Hospital Health Care Management

Hospital Health Care Management

C. Charles

ANMOL PUBLICATIONS PVT. LTD.
NEW DELHI - 110 002 (INDIA)

ANMOL PUBLICATIONS PVT. LTD.
H.O.: 4374/4B, Ansari Road, Daryaganj,
New Delhi-110 002 (India)
Ph.: 23278000, 23261597
B.O.: No. 1015, Ist Main Road, BSK IIIrd Stage
IIIrd Phase, IIIrd Block,
Bangalore - 560 085 (India)
Visit us at: www.anmolpublications.com

Hospital Health Care Management

First Published, 2008

ISBN 978-81-261-3288-1

PRINTED IN INDIA

Printed at Mehra Offset Press, Delhi.

Contents

Preface

Health status is considered as the state of health of a specified individual, group, or population. It may be measured by obtaining proxies such as people's subjective assessments of their health; by one or more indicators of mortality and morbidity in the population, such as longevity or maternal and infant mortality; or by using the incidence or prevalence of major diseases (communicable, chronic, or nutritional). Conceptually, health status is the proper outcome measure for the effectiveness of a specific population's medical care system, although attempts to relate effects of available medical care to variations in health status have proved difficult. Throughout the healthcare industry, improving the overall standard of patient care has become the primary aim of physicians, medical facilities and pharmaceutical suppliers worldwide. Vastly increased financial investment is proof of their commitment yet the achievement of this goal is complicated by both the need for operational efficiency and the demands of an increasing and ageing population. This reference publication provides an invaluable knowledge to physicians and healthcare professionals by examining and promoting the technologies – existing and emerging – that offer the best treatment options, while considering the logistical implications of delivering the highest possible standards of treatment. The hospital network is central to any mission of making quality healthcare services widely available to the community at large. From the network of recognized hospitals, one may accrue such tangible patient benefits, such as: a consistently high level of medical care;

access to a large pool of specialists with expertise across a vast spectrum of medical disciplines; patient information transfer if you were to move from one location to another, made possible by in-house IT connectivity, etc.

Health care clearinghouse is a public or private entity that does either of the following (Entities, including but not limited to, billing services, repricing companies, community health management information systems or community health information systems, and "value-added" networks and switches are health care clearinghouses if they perform these functions): 1) Processes or facilitates the processing of information received from another entity in a nonstandard format or containing nonstandard data content into standard data elements or a standard transaction; 2) Receives a standard transaction from another entity and processes or facilitates the processing of information into nonstandard format or nonstandard data content for a receiving entity. Health care operations includes institutional activities that are necessary to maintain and monitor the operations of the institution. Examples include but are not limited to: conducting quality assessment and improvement activities; developing clinical guidelines; case management; reviewing the competence or qualifications of health care professionals; education and training of students, trainees and practitioners; fraud and abuse programs; business planning and management; and customer service. Under the HIPAA Privacy Rule, these are allowable uses and disclosures of identifiable information "without specific authorization." Research is not considered part of health care operations. Health care providers are those providers of medical or health care or researchers who provide health care are health care providers. Normally health care providers are clinics, hospitals, doctors, dentists, psychologists and similar professionals. Similarly, Healthcare provider taxonomy code is an administrative code set that classifies health care providers by type and area of specialization. The code set will be used in certain adopted transactions.

Hospital healthcare system includes a wide array of programs and services. From robotic surgery and minimally invasive hip replacement to the latest in cancer treatment, Hospital healthcare system provides access to high quality., cost-effective health services. For example, the wide range of services may include: women's health; community cancer program; heart program; center for joint replacement; the institute for minimally invasive and robotic surgery; the sports medicine center; occupational medicine – well for work; hospital's program; other services; etc. The global healthcare sector continues to grow year on year, largely as a result of rising in-patient admissions, more intensive and expensive in-patient care and the growth of the hospital equipment expenditure. These factors mean healthcare providers are required to focus their efforts on improving the quality of care and information sharing whilst reducing costs and medical errors.

—Editor

1

Introduction to Health Needs and Health Care Plans & Programmes

PRIORITY HEALTH NEEDS

An assessment of Mississippi's health care system reveals gaps and unmet needs in several areas. The MSDH has identified the following priority health needs for Mississippi:

— Disease prevention, health protection, and health promotion

— Health care for specific populations, such as mothers, babies, the elderly, the indigent, the uninsured, and minorities

— Implementation of a statewide trauma system

— Health needs of persons with mental illness, alcohol/drug abuse problems, and/or mental retardation/developmental disabilities

— Availability of adequate health manpower throughout the state

— Enhanced capacity for detection of and response to public health emergencies, including acts of bioterrorism.

Health Care for Specific Populations

Mothers and Babies

Mississippi has high rates of infant mortality, low

birthweight, and teenage pregnancy. Contributing factors are late or inadequate prenatal care; unhealthy lifestyle factors such as inadequate prenatal nutrition, maternal smoking, or substance abuse; medical or congenital disorders; low socio-economic status; and low educational attainment. To combat these problems, the state must ensure that all persons receive the services necessary to prevent unplanned pregnancies and to promote healthy pregnancies and births. These services include:

- early health education to encourage teenagers to postpone sexual involvement;
- accessible family planning services to prevent unplanned pregnancies;
- comprehensive and risk-appropriate prenatal care, including medical, nursing, nutritional, educational, and social services, to ensure optimal pregnancy outcome;
- obstetrical delivery at a hospital appropriate for the level of patient risk involved; and
- regular pediatric assessments, timely childhood immunisations, and sick care for the infant to ensure a healthy start in life.

The MSDH provides maternity services state wide through county health departments, targeting pregnant women whose incomes are at or below 185 per cent of the federal poverty level. Since 1984, a Task Force on Infant Mortality has assisted the MSDH in developing strategies to prevent unintended pregnancies, encourage comprehensive prenatal care, implement regionalized perinatal services, and improve access to prenatal and delivery care. Improvements resulting from the efforts of this Task Force include the expansion of Medicaid eligibility for pregnant women and for infants and children; implementation of case management and enhanced services for high risk pregnant women and infants; development of a regionalized perinatal care system; and school nurse programmes. The MSDH also involves itself in special maternity/perinatal service initiatives, including a Perinatal High Risk Management/Infant Services System (PHRM/ISS) to reduce low birthweight and infant mortality through a comprehensive array of supplemental services. More information on these programmes.

In addition, the MSDH provides other programmes/ projects aimed at identifying contributing factors to infant mortality or factors that may lead to special developmental needs of an infant. These include:

— *Pregnancy Risk Assessment Monitoring System (PRAMS):* PRAMS is part of the Centers for Disease Control and Prevention initiative to reduce infant mortality and low birthweight. It is an ongoing, population-based, state-specific source of information on selected maternal behaviours and experiences that occur before and during pregnancy and during a child's early infancy.

— *Maternal and Infant Mortality Surveillance System (MIMS):* MIMs is a surveillance system through which maternal and infant death data are collected and reviewed. The purpose of these reviews is to understand how a wide array of local, social, economic, public health, educational, environmental, and safety issues relate to the tragedy of the loss.

— *Genetic Services:* These services include hemoglobinopathy services (screening, education, follow-up, and treatment); clinical genetics (genetics clinics, education, and treatment); newborn screening (recently expanded to include 40 genetic disorders);

Birth Defects Registry (birth defects database, registry, and tracking); and case management and provider education to more than 70 hospital nurseries, laboratories, and 120 health department clinics.

— *Early Hearing Detection and Intervention Program:* This programme is responsible for the universal new born hearing screening programme, including testing, diagnosis, tracking, and follow-up. Children identified through this programme as having a hearing loss are referred to the MSDH Early Intervention programme for services and follow-up.

Maternal and Child Health Five-Year Needs Assessment

Every five years, the Maternal and Child Health Bureau requires states to conduct a needs assessment to assure the appropriateness of each state's maternal and child health (MCH) services. The MCH staff is currently developing the needs assessments for FY 2005. The Title V MCH Needs Assessment Report 2000 creates a composite picture of the maternal and child health population in Mississippi. It describes the emerging needs of the population and the changes in the larger health care system which have occurred since the previous needs assessment in 1995. The report identifies the need for preventive and primary care services for pregnant women, mothers, and infants; preventive and primary care services for children, including adolescents; and services for children with special health care needs.

The current five-year needs assessment reflects numerous needs for women, infants, children, adolescents, and children with special health care needs. The following is a list of priorities selected and prioritized as a means of improving the status of maternal and child health services in Mississippi as a result of the MCH needs assessment:

— Reduce repeat teen births;

— Improve data collection capacity for Title V populations;
— Explore coverage of asthma services for children;
— Increase EPSDT screening among children on Medicaid;
— Reduce the state's low birthweight rate and infant mortality rate;
— Develop a plan to identify, gather data on, and address issues related to maternal deaths;
— Decrease cigarette smoking among ninth through twelfth graders;
— Decrease the incidence of teen mortality and unhealthy behaviours;
— Assure access to pediatric care for all children, including children with special health care needs; and
— Decrease cigarette smoking among pregnant adolescents.

A new five-year assessment will be completed by 2005.

Disease Prevention, Health Protection, and Health Promotion

Many of the health problems that plague Mississippians are the result of the state's social, economic, and educational conditions. Mississippi has the second lowest per capita and family income in the nation. Information from the 2000 U.S. Census showed that the state ranks below the national average in the percentage of its population who are high school graduates and college graduates. Mississippi continues to lead the nation in infant death rate, teenage pregnancy, births to unwed mothers, and sexually transmitted diseases (especially syphilis). However, with the state's improved economic situation, many of these problems are being aggressively addressed. Ten leading causes resulted in 80.4 percent of all deaths in Mississippi during 2002. Lifestyle choices are a contributing factor to many of the leading causes of death; most of the premature death, injury, and disability in Mississippi is related to only six risk factors: tobacco use, poor diet, sedentary lifestyle, intentional and unintentional injury, drug and alcohol abuse, and sexual behaviour.

Early detection and prevention efforts can greatly influence other factors. For example, a screening and treatment programme for hypertension can help avoid some of the costs associated with premature death and disability due to heart disease and stroke. Other prominent factors contributing to heart disease and stroke are cigarette smoking, elevated blood cholesterol levels, diabetes, and obesity. Almost all of these factors can be averted with proper preventive measures.

Prevention costs significantly less than managing disease or disability. Mississippi's high rates of mortality and morbidity in many areas cause high costs for health and social services. Properly directed and increased expenditures for such preventive services as prenatal care, family planning services, cardiovascular disease prevention, targeted screening, and health education could help avoid greater expenditures in the future from premature births, teenage pregnancies, heart disease, stroke, accidents, tuberculosis, sexually transmitted diseases (including HIV/AIDS), and other problems. Continued and increased support in disease prevention and health promotion is a cost effective approach toward improving the health status of Mississippians.

The MSDH maintains numerous programmes directed toward disease prevention and health promotion. For example, its Office of Epidemiology provides a statewide surveillance programme to monitor and investigate the occurrence and trends of reportable diseases and provides consultation to health care professionals and the public on communicable disease control and prevention. The immunisation programme provides and supports services designed to ultimately eliminate morbidity and mortality due to childhood vaccine-preventable diseases. The HIV/AIDS prevention and sexually transmitted disease programmes offer treatment and drug counseling, testing, and referral services. The Office of Health Promotion directs activities in areas such as injury/violence prevention and control, physical activity, worksite health promotion, cardiovascular disease and diabetes prevention and control, school health, community health promotion, and tobacco prevention and cessation. In addition, the Mississippi Legislature has authorized a Mississippi Council on Obesity Prevention and Management and a Task Force on Heart Disease and Stroke Prevention. With the assistance of the Department of Health, these groups will develop a comprehensive statewide plan to address each of these critical public health problems. The MSDH is also developing state plans related to arthritis and diabetes in Mississippi.

The Elderly

Although the majority of the state's younger elderly persons remain relatively healthy, general health and mobility decline with advancing years. About 25 per cent of persons aged 85 or older cannot perform the essential activities of daily living. These "frail elderly" persons require nursing home care or extensive medical and social support in the home. However, few elderly persons can afford extended long-term care. Societal trends in the United States have produced smaller family units and fewer unemployed family members, making the option of home care by the family of elderly persons less available than in past years. Financing for physician care and medication becomes more difficult for the elderly as Medicare deductibles and co-insurance payments increase.

Home health services play an important role in providing needed health care for the homebound elderly, but the care is provided on an intermittent basis and is limited to skilled rehabilitative care. Most elderly people lack adequate financing for custodial care, leaving nursing home care as the only option for many. Medicaid is the primary payor for this expensive care; however, Medicaid has strict limits on the amount of income and assets a person may have and still receive assistance. In addition, the Legislature has limited the number of nursing home beds allowed to participate in the Medicaid programme because of the tremendous cost of nursing home care.

The state must continue to examine ways to expand health care services for the elderly population. The Legislature has authorized expansion of current and creation of new home and community-based waiver programmes through the Division of Medicaid. These programmes are designed to allow Medicaid eligible individuals to avoid or delay institutionalisation. The Division operates five waiver programmes; two are specifically designed to assist elderly Mississippians: the Elderly Disabled Waiver and the Assisted Living Waiver. Services available through these waiver programmes include case management, expanded home health, homemaker, adult day health, home delivered meals, escorted transportation, and in-home and institutional respite. The MSDH endorses the continuing development of residential retirement communities, supervised living apartments, assisted living facilities, personal care homes, adult day care centers, respite care services, and home and community-based services. The MSDH encourages all skilled nursing homes participating in the Medicaid programme to also participate in Medicare, supports the funding of a broad spectrum of senior citizen services, and recommends the limited expansion of nursing home beds in the state according to the statistical formula for Certificate of Need.

Minorities

Advances in technology, medication, treatment, and disease management have led to marked improvements in the health and longevity of Americans. However, gaps between the health status of whites and nonwhites continue to show disturbing disparities. Reducing or eliminating such risk factors as smoking, improper nutrition, and substance abuse would decrease morbidity and mortality rates in the minority community. One or more of these factors contribute to all the conditions causing excess mortality among minority populations. Other factors include lack of early identification of disease, lack of access to health care, and poverty. Moreover, programmes designed to reduce or eliminate high risk behaviours have more significantly benefitted the majority population.

Many of the factors contributing to excess deaths in the state's minority population are related to lifestyle. This situation emphasizes the need for health promotion and disease prevention within the minority community. The black male faces the greatest disparity in health indicators. He is more likely to die young, and the cause of death is usually homicide. Answers must be found to mitigate or stop the increase of black male homicide/violence. Barriers to adequate health care for minorities include lack of access to the health care system, the cultural insensitivity of providers, and the lack of health insurance services. Possible solutions include promoting health education for providers (especially minority providers), funding services and programmes targeted to minorities, and evaluating the effectiveness of programmes that minority groups need.

After receiving input from various citizens groups residing in Mississippi, the Mississippi State Department of Health developed a comprehensive plan to address the health problems unique to minority groups of the state, specifically African Americans. African Americans are the primary ethnic group statistically impacting Mississippi at this time; however, other racial and ethnic minorities are not ignored. The Plan can be used as a baseline for improvement of health care practices as other ethnic groups migrate to the state in larger numbers. The Plan, entitled Plan to Eliminate Racal and Ethnic Health Care Disparities, identifies poverty, the influx of large minority groups, lower educational levels, and limited health manpower, particularly in rural areas, as conditions that contribute to racial and ethnic health care disparities. The Plan emphasizes cardiovascular disease, diabetes, cancer screening, HIV/AIDS, child/adult immunisation, and infant mortality as six areas of health care disparities most often experienced by minority groups at all life stages.

After health care data was collected and evaluated, five issues emerged as methods to eliminate health care disparities in multiple racial and ethnic minority groups. These issues include cultural competency, prevention/education, accessibility/availability, funding/finance, and legislation. The Plan addresses strategies, action steps, and desired outcomes. Strategies include the creation of partnerships to provide health insurance coverage, increasing the number of under-represented minorities in health professions, increasing the number of consumers on healthcare provider boards, increasing community health education outreach activities of hospital and health care agencies, and preparing health and human service professionals for patient cross-cultural relationships. Action steps to facilitate these strategies include creating partnerships with other state agencies, faith-based agencies, community-based organisations, and provider groups to strengthen the ability to fully serve and effectively address the health care needs of all citizens in the state.

The Indigent and Uninsured

The traditional sources of reimbursement for indigent care have not kept pace with the increased number of indigent patients, and some traditional sources have diminished. Two undesirable events occur as a result of these circumstances: (1) indigent persons delay or forego needed health care, resulting in increased morbidity and mortality; and 2) health care providers deliver increased amounts of uncompensated care, resulting in severe financial distress for providers who serve significant numbers of indigent patients. The medically indigent population is comprised of several groups of people:

— unemployed or self-employed persons with no health insurance;
— employees of small businesses and agencies which do not provide health insurance;
— part-time employees who are not eligible for health insurance;
— persons covered by insurance and in need of services not covered by insurance; and
— the uninsured and under-insured non-poor who experience high costs due to catastrophic illness.

The working poor who earn too much to qualify for Medicaid and who are not provided health insurance benefits by their employer are financially unable to purchase needed primary care services and create serious uncompensated care problems for service providers. Small rural hospitals, serving populations comprised of a large proportion of uninsured or under-insured individuals, are struggling to survive financially. The cost of uncompensated care, shifted to the bills of paying patients, has doubled since 1980. The American Hospital Association estimates that about 16 percent is added to every medical bill of patients with private insurance to help defray the cost of indigent health care. However, hospitals are finding it increasingly more difficult to shift these costs. The largest health care customers — American businesses and industries through employee health insurance policies — have demanded discounts and lower prices. Additionally, as the organisation and structure of health care delivery has changed from a cost-based reimbursement to a uniform prospective payment system, healthcare providers (particularly hospitals) are finding it difficult to continue traditional charity care for an increasing indigent population. The high cost of uninsured health care bankrupts families as well. The elderly person who needs long-term care for a chronic illness is financially impoverished before Medicaid reimbursement becomes available. The young couple with a chronically ill child may face tremendous financial burdens and live on the edge of poverty to pay for care for their uninsurable child.

This situation also creates serious health problems for the individual. The Medicare recipient who receives a minimal Social Security payment must often decide between buying food or medicine and frequently forgoes essential health care. Uninsured individuals with chronic diseases cannot afford prescribed medication and therefore do not properly manage their illness. A pregnant woman delays prenatal care and thus endangers both her health and that of her unborn child. While there are no precise measures of the number of Mississippians who have been refused health care, or of the amount of charity care provided, there are some useful indicators of the extent of medical indigence, including the number of persons who have no health insurance. Nationally, about 17 percent of the non-elderly population has no health insurance. Approximately 518,000 or 22.1 percent of the non-elderly population in Mississippi has no health insurance, according to the Employee Benefit Research Institute.

Implementation of a Statewide Trauma System

Trauma is the leading cause of death for all age groups in Mississippi from birth to age 44. Serious injury and death resulting from trauma events such as vehicle crashes, falls, and firearms claim 2,000 lives and disable 6,000 Mississippians each year. Trauma victims require immediate, expert attention. Following the recommendations of a Trauma Care Task Force, the Mississippi Legislature gave the MSDH authority to develop a statewide trauma care system and established a permanent trust fund to finance the system. The Trauma Care Trust Fund receives funding through a $5 assessment on all moving traffic violations. The fund provides administrative functions at both the state and regional levels.

The Mississippi Legislature added $6 million to the Trauma Care Trust Fund during the 1999 session, increasing the annual Trust Fund to approximately $8 million. Funds are available for designated Trauma Care Regions through annual contracts with the MSDH Bureau of EMS. The fund is divided between designated trauma center hospitals and eligible physicians on an allocation of 70 percent to hospitals and 30 percent to physicians. During 2002, a total allocation of $7,030,454 was distributed to 70 hospitals and 314 surgeons for trauma care. The MSDH has designated seven trauma care regions; each is incorporated as a 501c-3organisation and contracts with the MSDH to develop and implement a Regional Trauma Plan. The Mississippi Trauma Care System Plan received approval in October 2002 and includes the seven regional trauma plans. The plan allows for trauma patients to be transported to the "most appropriate" trauma facility for their injuries.

Designation levels set specific criteria and standards of care that guide hospital and emergency personnel in determining the level of care a trauma victim needs and whether that hospital can care for the patient or transfer the patient to a Trauma Center that can administer more definitive care.

Level I Trauma Centers must have a full range of trauma capabilities, including an emergency department, a full-service surgical suite, intensive care unit, and diagnostic imaging. Level I Centers must have a residency programme, ongoing trauma research, and provide 24-hour trauma service. These hospitals provide a variety of other services to comprehensively care for both trauma patients and medical patients. Level I Trauma Centers act as referral facilities for Level II, III, and IV Trauma Centers.

Level II Trauma Centers must be able to provide initial care to the severely injured patient. These facilities must have a full range of trauma capabilities, including an emergency department, a full service surgical suite, an intensive care unit, and diagnostic imaging. Level II Trauma Centers act as referral facilities for Level III and IV Trauma Centers. For specialty care a patient may be transferred to a Level I Trauma Center.

Level III Trauma Centers must offer continuous general surgical coverage and have the ability to manage the initial care of many injured patients. Level III Trauma Centers must also provide continuous orthopedic coverage. Transfer agreements must be in place with Level I and II Trauma Centers for patients that exceed the Level III Trauma Center's resources. Level III centers may act as referral facilities for Level IV Trauma Centers.

Level IV Trauma Centers provide initial evaluation and assessment of injured patients. Most patients will require transfer to facilities with more resources dedicated to providing optimal care for the injured patients. Level IV Trauma Centers must have transfer agreements in place with Level I, II, and III Trauma Centers.

Mississippi Trauma Care Regions

North Mississippi Trauma Care Region, Inc. serves an 18-county area in the northeast portion of the state, encompassing 8,777 square miles. Counties include: Alcorn, Benton, Choctaw, Clay, Chickasaw, Calhoun, Itawamba, Lee, Lafayette, Lowndes, Oktibbeha, Monroe, Pontotoc, Prentiss, Tippah, Tishomingo, Union, and Webster. There are 18 hospitals in the Region; 17 hospitals with emergency rooms are participating in the Mississippi Trauma Care System. The region has one fully designated Level IV hospital – Tippah County Hospital, Ripley, and two Level II hospitals - North Mississippi Medical Center, Tupelo, and Baptist Memorial Hospital/Golden Triangle, Columbia.

Delta Mississippi Trauma Care Region, Inc. serves a 19-county area in the west central portion of the state, encompassing 10,518 square miles. Counties include: DeSoto, Tunica, Tate, Marshall, Coahoma, Quitman, Panola, Bolivar, Sunflower, Tallahatchie, Yalobusha, Grenada, Leflore, Washington, Humphreys, Carroll, Montgomery, Sharkey, and Issaquena. There are a total of 19 hospitals in the Region; 16 hospitals with emergency rooms are participating in the Mississippi Trauma Care System. Central Mississippi Trauma Care Region serves a 14-county, 9,616 square mile area in the westcentral portion of the state. Counties include: Attala, Claiborne, Copiah, Hinds, Holmes, Jefferson, Leake, Madison, Rankin, Scott, Simpson, Smith, Warren and Yazoo. The Region contains a total of 21 hospitals; 14 hospitals with emergency rooms are participating in the Mississippi Trauma Care System. The region has two fully designated Level IV hospitals– Rankin Medical Center, Brandon, and Scott Regional Hospital, Morton, and one Level I hospital - The University Hospital and Clinics, Jackson.

East Central Mississippi Trauma Care Region serves a seven-county area in the eastern portion of the state, including: Winston, Noxubee, Neshoba, Kemper, Newton, Lauderdale, and Clarke. There are a total of 10 hospitals with emergency rooms that are participating in the Mississippi Trauma Care System. Southwest Mississippi Trauma Care Region serves a seven-county area in the southwest portion of the state. Counties include: Adams, Franklin, Wilkinson, Amite, Lincoln, Pike and Lawrence. There are a total of eight hospitals with emergency rooms participating in the Mississippi Trauma Care System. Lawrence County Hospital, a Level IV center, is the region's sole trauma center. Southeast Mississippi Trauma Care Region serves a 13-county area in the southeastern portion of the state. Counties include: Covington, Forrest, Greene, Jasper, Jones, Lamar, Perry, Pearl River, Walthall, Marion, Wayne, Stone, and Jefferson Davis. There are 12 hospitals in this region, with ten participating in the Mississippi Trauma Care System. This region has a fully designated Level II trauma center - Forrest General Hospital in Hattiesburg, a Level III trauma center-South Central Regional Medical Center in Laurel, and two Level IV trauma centers - Wayne General Hospital in Waynesboro and L.O. Crosby Memorial Hospital in Picayune. Coastal Mississippi Trauma Care Region serves four counties in the southern portion of the state: Jackson, Harrison, Hancock, and George. Seven hospitals participate in the Mississippi Trauma Care System. Presently, Gulf Coast Medical Center in Biloxi has been designated as a Level III Trauma Center, and Ocean Springs Hospital in Pascagoula as a Level IV Center. In total, 91 per cent of Mississippi hospitals with an emergency room are part of the Mississippi Trauma Care System.

Health Needs of Persons with Mental Illness, Alcohol/Drug Abuse Problems, and/or Mental Retardation/ Developmental Disabilities

Access to a full range of care for persons with mental illness or alcohol/drug abuse problems could prove difficult. State government provides or finances the majority of mental health services, particularly residential treatment services. Mississippi has made a considerable investment in mental health facilities and services, and the state has a number of private sector facilities; yet, a substantial number of Mississippians cannot obtain needed mental health care. The high cost and limited third party coverage of private sector mental health services denies access to all but the wealthy or persons with exceptional health insurance coverage. Efforts to improve access include additional facilities opened or under construction by the Mississippi Department of Mental Health; an increase in the number of group homes for persons with chronic mental illness, operated by state hospitals or regional mental health/mental retardation centers; and the opening of group homes for emotionally disturbed children to prevent institutional placement or to provide a placement for adolescents ready for discharge from the state hospital.

The existing triad of the Department of Mental Health, regional community mental health/mental retardation centers, and private sector providers has the potential of supporting a comprehensive network capable of providing vitally needed services for persons with mental illness or mental retardation. Mississippi Access to Care (MAC), a statewide initiative to assess and respond to the needs of individuals with disabilities, began in the fall of 2000. Participating in this initiative are persons with disabilities and their family members; service providers; associations; advocates; state agencies, including the Departments of Education, Health, Human Services, Mental Health, Rehabilitation Services, and the Division of Medicaid; local agencies; and any other persons or organisations interested in making the greatest possible independence available to those with disabilities. The MAC work group developed a written comprehensive plan which was submitted to the Legislature in October 2001 and considered during the 2002 session. The intent of the plan was to address the needs of persons with disabilities and their families and identify possibilities for bringing the goal of greater independence within closer reach.

First Steps Early Intervention Programme (FSEIP) is Mississippi's early intervention system for infants and toddlers with special developmental needs and their families. First Steps is implemented through an interagency system of comprehensive developmental services for eligible infants andtoddlers. The statewide system seeks to minimize the impact of a disabling condition on an infant or toddler and his or her family by identifying and utilizing community-based resources to the maximum extent possible. The process of connecting an eligible infant to the provision of services and transition of toddlers into an appropriate educational setting is well orchestrated in keeping with the regulations of the Individuals with Disabilities Education Act (IDEA) Part C. Mississippi serves all eligible infants and toddlers and their families. The programme provides child find, procedural safeguards, service coordination, evaluation and assessment, and transition services free of charge to families. After a comprehensive, multi-disciplinary evaluation and assessment, specialized developmental services may be provided to the child and family in accordance with an individualized family service plan (IFSP). All services are currently provided at no cost to families. Cost for specialized developmental services may be charged to private insurance or Medicaid. If the family has no form of insurance coverage, the MSDH as the lead agency may pay for services as "payor of last resort."

Availability of Adequate Health Manpower

Essential health service delivery requires an adequate supply and appropriate distribution of fully qualified physicians, nurses, and other health care personnel. Mississippi has an adequate total of physicians to meet national standards; however, the physicians are maldistributed through the state. As of July 2004, 65 counties or portions of counties were designated as health professional shortage areas for primary medical care. Mississippi needs to further encourage the training of primary care physicians who will practice in designated underserved areas. Consideration should be given to using community hospitals more extensively for residency training in family medicine.

Approximately 40 percent of Mississippi's dentists practice in the two major metropolitan areas: Jackson and the Gulf Coast. The state's goal is to improve the distribution of dentists so that no county has more than 5,000 persons per dentist and primary dental care is available within 30 minutes travel time of all areas. The Mississippi Nurses' Association (MNA) and 25 nursing organisations are working together through the MNA's Nursing Organisation Liaison Committee to address nursing manpower issues related to anticipated changes in the workplace. Through the efforts of this group, the Mississippi Legislature authorized an Office of Nursing Workforce to develop a statewide model for predicting nursing manpower needs and to initiate methods of transitioning nurses as needed from jobs in the acute care setting to jobs in the community.

The supply of allied health professionals has increased in recent years, with the work force distributed to virtually all health care settings. Firm conclusions about the supply and demand for allied health personnel are difficult to draw, because very little data is available for the study of these groups of health professionals. However, officials believe that changes in the health care delivery system, the aging of the population, and advances in health service techniques and technology will continue to increase the demand for qualified technologists and technicians. In addition, the U.S. Health Resources and Services Administration (HRSA) supports the development of systems to improve access to preventive and primary care by providing funding, human resources, and technical assistance to states and community-based organisations. To support state efforts, funds are provided for cooperative agreements to maintain a Primary Care Office (PCO) in each of the 50 states, the District of Columbia, and Puerto Rico.

The Mississippi State Department of Health has housed a PCO for more than 18 years. The programme is responsible for primary care needs assessment and plan development, health manpower recruitment, coordination of National Health Service Corps and foreign-trained providers, developing linkages with health professional schools, Health Professional Shortage Area designations, researching health care disparities, and assisting in marketplace analysis for primary care delivery sites.

The PCO also assists in coordination of primary care

services by working with Federally Qualified Community Health Centers and other organisations to help place physicians in underserved areas. The PCO administers and/ or makes recommendations regarding the placement of foreign medical graduates through the J-1 Visa waiver programmes. Through these programmes, an exchange visitor can be granted a waiver of the two-year foreign residence requirement of the Immigration and Nationality Act if their stay is in the public interest and they agree to serve in underserved areas. There are currently 86 foreign providers actively practicing in Mississippi – 17 placed through the Appalachian Regional Commission, 69 placed through the State 20/30 Programme, and one through the Delta Regional Authority.

The PCO also assists the National Health Service Corps (NHSC) in the placement of healthcare professionals – primary care physicians, dentists, nurse practitioners, and psychiatrists – in health professional shortage areas through loan repayment and scholarship programmes. The current NHSC field strength is 53 and growing as a result of President Bush's Management for Growth initiative. The NHSC seeks to improve the health of underserved Americans by bringing quality primary health care professionals to communities in need, as well as supporting communities in their efforts to build better systems of care. Public Health Preparedness and Response for Emergencies. In 1998, the Centers for Disease Control began providing funds to state departments of health to prepare for and respond to bioterrorism. Since then, the Mississippi State Department of Health has used those funds to improve the capabilities of the Department to respond to all public heath emergencies, including bioterrorism. Following the events of September 2001 and the subsequent anthrax incidents that affected the nation, Congress approved an unprecedented increase in funding for public health to combat bioterrorism and improve the public health infrastructure of the nation. Every state received money in seven emphasis areas to improve response efforts. Mississippi's response efforts are based on the overarching principal that all response is local. In essence, the response begins before the threat is fully recognized, emphasizing the need for a well-trained, well-coordinated response plan. The following outline represents the basic response plans and efforts based on the areas of emphasis as identified by the CDC.

Preparedness Planning focuses on the Department's ability to respond to all emergencies, including acts of bioterrorism. For the first time, the Department has had the opportunity to position emergency response coordinators in each district, with the direct responsibility of strengthening ties with the community and helping integrate public health into local emergency response efforts. Further, this emphasis area highlights readiness assessment, which the Department will use to identify deficiencies in the response system and to make plans for future improvements.

Surveillance and Epidemiological Capacity has been greatly enhanced with the funding from this grant. Both technological and human resources have been enhanced to improve surveillance activities and move toward a "real time" reporting system, the National Electronic Disease Surveillance System (NEDSS). NEDSS is being implemented in association with the bioterrorism programme to link Mississippi to a national reporting system and improve response efforts beyond the state. Many of the grant activities proved invaluable in implementing the Department's small pox vaccination programme, and will continue to provide increased coverage to combat emerging public health issues such as West Nile Virus and Severe Acute Respiratory Syndrome (SARS).

Laboratory Capacity has been enhanced in two separate areas: Biological Agents and Chemical Agents. While the Chemical Agent funding is new for the 2003-2004 funding cycle, the Biological Agents funding has already greatly improved laboratory capacity to respond in testing for agents such as anthrax, and has provided much-needed equipment and staff. The Public Health Laboratory (PHL) has been able to implement a coordinated training programme for other laboratories statewide, and has added a molecular biology section to the lab. One of the biggest problems facing the PHL at this time is finding space to conduct the tests; that problem is going to be solved, in part, with installation of a modular unit later this year. That unit will be necessary to further increase lab capacity to test chemical agents.

The *Health Alert Network* is responsible for providing accurate, timely health alerts and information to appropriate audiences through secure channels. Building on systems already in place in the surveillance programme, the MS-HAN plans to upgrade alerting capabilities to include the ability to provide health alert messages via multiple channels to physicians, emergency rooms, infection control specialists, and non-traditional partners in law enforcement, emergency response, and fire departments. Further, the system will integrate with other information systems as part of the Public Health Information Network (PHIN), which includes HAN, NEDSS, the Laboratory Response Network (LRN), and other CDC-sponsored efforts.

Risk Communication and Health Information Dissemination focuses on the Department's ability to communicate high-risk and highly technical information to both the media and the public. Communications with the media focus on clear, concise messages prepared and delivered by public health professionals trained in media relations.

Information for the public includes general information regarding bioterrorism and other public health emergencies, including emerging infectious diseases. The grant funding has allowed the Department to upgrade and expand the web site capabilities, providing a more streamlined and user-friendly vehicle for both public communication and services.

Education and Training are the foundation for preparing any team for response efforts. Through this grant, the Department plans to work toward a comprehensive, cohesive training plan for employees with an emphasis on workforce development and emergency response. Creation of a Learning Management System which links to a national system and gives employees the opportunity to select training is planned, as well as strengthening existing partnerships within the South Central Public Health group, a consortium which includes the state health departments in Mississippi, Louisiana, Alabama, and Arkansas, and the Schools of Public Health at the Tulane University School of Public Health and Tropical Medicine and the University of Alabama at Birmingham. Through all of these emphasis areas, the grant funding has emphasized improving ties between MSDH and communities, and improving the practice of public health in Mississippi. In addition, the U.S. Department of Health and Human Services Health Resources and Services Administration began funding in 2002 for a Bioterrorism Hospital Preparedness programme. The MSDH Office of Emergency Planning and Response administers this programme through its Bureau of Emergency Preparedness. The programme is to develop, implement, and intensify regional terrorism preparedness plans and protocols for hospitals, outpatient facilities, EMS systems (both free standing and fire-based), and poison control centers in a collaborative statewide and regional model.

Surge capacity has been addressed by forming seven emergency preparedness regions; each can address a surge capacity of at least 500 patients presenting as a direct result of bioterrorism, weapons of mass destruction, or other public health emergency. Specific hospitals in each region have been identified as Weapons of Mass Destruction Centers of Excellence. Each of these preparedness-enhanced facilities are receiving pharmaceutical caches, personal protective equipment, decontamination units, communication upgrades, isolation capability upgrades, and training. Emergency medical services, hospitals, and hospital laboratories will receive benefits as well, including communications improvements, training in planning and response, personal protective equipment, and pharmaceutical caches.

MANAGED HEALTH CARE PLANS

What is Managed Health Care?

It's a system that controls the financing and delivery of health services to members who are enrolled in a specific type of healthcare plan. The goals of managed health care are to ensure that:

— providers deliver high-quality care in an environment that manages or controls costs.

— the care delivered is medically necessary and appropriate for the patient's condition.

— care is rendered by the most appropriate provider.

— care is rendered in the most appropriate, least-restrictive setting.

What are the Major Types of Managed Care Plans?

— Health Maintenance Organisations (HMO)

— Preferred Provider Organisations (PPO)

— Point-of-Service (POS) plans

Each of these systems has distinctive features or characteristics.

Health Maintenance Organisations (HMO)

— An HMO enters into contractual arrangements with healthcare providers (e.g., physicians, hospitals and other healthcare professionals) who together form a "provider network." In simple terms, a contracted provider is one who provides services to health plan members at discounted rates in exchange for receiving health plan referrals.

— Members are required to see only providers within this network to have their healthcare paid for by the HMO. If the member receives care from a provider who isn't in the network, the HMO won't pay for care unless it was pre-authorized by the HMO or deemed an emergency.

— Members select a Primary Care Physician (PCP), often called a "gatekeeper," who provides, arranges, coordinates and authorizes all aspects of the member's health care. PCPs are usually family doctors, internal medicine doctors, general practitioners and obstetricians/gynecologists.

— Members can only see a specialist (e.g., cardiologist, dermatologist, rheumatologist) if this is authorized by the PCP. If the member sees a specialist without a referral, the HMO won't pay for the care.

— HMOs are the most restrictive type of health plan because they give members the least choice in selecting a health care provider. However, HMOs typically provide members with a greater range of health benefits for the lowest out-of-pocket expenses, such as either no or a very low copayment (the amount of money a member is required to pay the provider in addition to what the HMO pays. It often must be paid prior to services being rendered).

Preferred Provider Organisations (PPO)

— PPOs are similar to HMOs in that they enter into contractual arrangements with healthcare providers (e.g., physicians, hospitals and other healthcare professionals) who together form a "provider network."

— Unlike an HMO, members don't have a PCP ("gatekeeper") nor do they have to use an in-network provider for their care. However, PPOs offer members "richer" benefits as financial incentives to use network providers. The incentives may include lower deductibles, lower co-payments and higher reimbursements. For example, if you see an in-network family physician for a routine visit, you may only have a small co-payment or deductible. If you see a non-network family physician for a routine visit, you may have to pay as much as 50 percent of the total bill.

— PPO members typically don't have to get a referral to see a specialist. However, as mentioned above, there's a financial incentive to use a specialist on the PPO's provider network.

— PPOs are less restrictive than HMOs in the choice of health care provider. However, they tend to require greater "out-of-pocket" payments from the members.

Point-of-Service Plans (POS)

— A POS plan is often called an HMO/PPO hybrid or an "open-ended" HMO. The reason it's called "point-of-service" is that members choose which option – HMO or PPO—they will use each time they seek health care.

— Like an HMO and a PPO, a POS plan has a contracted provider network.

— POS plans encourage, but don't require, members to choose a primary care physician (PCP). As in a traditional HMO, the PCP acts as a "gatekeeper" when making referrals. Members who choose not to use their PCPs for referrals (but still seek care from an in-network provider) still receive benefits but will pay higher copays and/or deductibles than members who use their PCPs.

— POS members also may opt to visit an out-of-network provider at their discretion. If so, a member copays, and coinsurance and deductibles are substantially higher.

— POS plans are becoming more popular because they offer more flexibility and freedom of choice than standard HMOs.

2

Health Care Financing and Delivery

DEVELOPMENT IN HEALTH CARE FINANCING AND DELIVERY

Health care financing and delivery arrangements have undergone dramatic changes in the past several decades. This section provides a brief overview of some of these developments, including changes in provider payment, the rise of managed care, and the integration (and then partial dis-integration) of health care delivery.

The Managed Care Backlash

Managed care grew so unpopular by the late-1990s that most commentators began referring to a "managed care backlash." Providers complained about the second-guessing of their clinical judgment, and argued that managed care undermined the doctor-patient relationship and quality of care. Consumers expressed concern that managed care was restricting choices, limiting access to necessary medical care, and lowering quality. Consumers were also exceedingly skeptical about the use of direct financial incentives and utilisation review. These concerns resulted in a substantial number of state and federal legislative and regulatory initiatives targeting more restrictive forms of managed care, along with private litigation. These initiatives have affected the forms of managed care available in the marketplace, although some commentators believe that competitive responses to the backlash had a bigger impact. Several commentators have argued that there is a substantial gap between consumer and provider perceptions and the actual impact of managed care. These commentators point to surveys and studies which show that consumers are generally satisfied with their own MCOs, that MCOs do not provide worse quality care than FFS medicine, and that managed care "horror stories" are often exaggerated or highly unrepresentative. Regardless, as Part C reflects, less restrictive forms of managed care have become extremely popular in recent years.

Fee for Service Reimbursement and the Rise of Managed Care

For most of the twentieth century, most consumers relied on independent physicians to provide care. Pricing was fee-for-service (FFS). FFS payment was based on the number and type of services performed. Insurers imposed few constraints on consumer choice of providers and limited oversight of the type and extent of care provided. FFS payment provided little incentive for physicians and other health care providers to coordinate and integrate the care they rendered. FFS arrangements conformed with public sentiment that more care was better care, and the treating physician was best positioned to judge the most appropriate care for any given case. Policy-makers began seriously questioning the consequences of these institutional arrangements in the late-1960s. Commentators argued that the combination of FFS payment, health insurance, and consumers' imperfect information about health care limited the possibility of effective price competition and created an incentive for physicians to over-provide (and consumers to over-consume) healthcare resources. Some commentators argued that organisations that agreed to meet the health care needs of a consumer for a set time period at a set price could solve these problems. More generally, many commentators argued that consumers should be given greater control over health care spending and treatment decisions.Over the past three decades, state and federal policy has encouraged the emergence of a range of financing and delivery options, and embraced, to varying degrees, price and non-price competition in health care.

Managed care existed for most of the 20 century, but it did not spread widely until the 1980s and early 1990s. In 1980, the overwhelming majority of the population was enrolled in an indemnity insurance plan and managed care organisations (MCOs) accounted for a small percentage of the market. Fifteen years later, these patterns had reversed, and various managed care offerings accounted for an overwhelming majority of the insured population. To be sure, managed care means different things to different people, and it has meant different things at different times. Commentators generally agree, however, that MCOs integrate, to varying degrees, the financing and delivery of health care services. Managed care encompasses a wide array of institutional arrangements for the financing and delivery of health care services. Usually when one speaks of a managed care organisation, one is speaking of the entity that manages risk, contracts with providers, is paid by employers or patient groups, or handles claims processing. The "tools" of managed care include the creation of networks of preferred providers or the hiring of a staff of employed physicians to provide care, selective contracting based on price, required pre-authorisation, restricted access to specialists, restricted panels of providers, higher copayments (and sometimes denial of coverage) for out-of-network care, capitation, bonuses, practice guidelines, retrospective denials of coverage, "real-time" utilisation review, restricted coverage of prescription drugs, disease management for chronic illnesses, limitations on benefits, and an emphasis on prevention.

In global terms, managed care offers a more restricted choice of (and access to) providers and treatments in exchange for lower premiums, deductibles, and co-payments than traditional indemnity insurance. Stated differently, managed care inverts, to varying degrees, the incentives of a piece-work based fee-for-service system, and employs a variety of supply- and demand-side strategies to do so. MCOs typically use three strategies to control costs and enhance quality of care: (i) selective contracting; (ii) direct financial incentives; and (iii) utilisation review. Selective contracting is used to create a restricted networks of providers. Selective contracting intensifies price competition and allows payors to negotiate volume discounts and choose providers based on a range of criteria. The intensity of competition increases with the number of providers and covered lives in the relevant market, and with the restrictiveness of the insurance contracts found in the market *(i.e.,* HMOs, which have more limited panels than PPOs, induce more intense price competition among providers than would PPOs of equivalent size).

When insurers have a credible threat to exclude providers from their networks and channel patients elsewhere, providers have a powerful incentive to bid aggressively. Inclusion in a restricted panel offers the provider the prospect of substantially increased revenue. Without such credible threats, however, providers have less incentive to bid aggressively, and even managed care organisations with large market shares may have less ability to obtain low prices. Direct financial incentives can take a variety of forms, including capitation, putting the physician on salary, and paying a bonus (or withholding a percentage of payment) based on meeting clinical and/or financial targets. Capitation pays the provider a fixed amount for each of the patients for whom he agrees to provide care, regardless of whether those patients seek care. Payment is typically based on a set number of dollars "per member-per month." In the mid-1990s, many commentators believed that capitation would become the basis for compensating most providers. Capitation lost some of its allure when some physician groups that had received capitation payments underestimated the associated costs, and were forced to file bankruptcy. Payors also grew less interested in capitation in the late-1990s, as providers became increasingly reluctant to accept the associated risks. Financial incentives can also be employed to encourage consumers to receive care from particular providers or in particular locations. Co-payments and deductibles are well-recognized forms of demand management.

Utilisation review appraises the appropriateness and medical necessity of the proposed treatment. Utilisation review can be conducted on a retrospective, concurrent, or prospective basis. Although many payors use utilisation review, the variety of forms it takes limit the ability to draw general conclusions about its effectiveness. These strategies can have an effect beyond the consumers covered by the MCO if providers tend to adopt a unitary standard of practice. Providers who must comply with certain quality protocols or report their performance for their MCO patients may (whether consciously or unconsciously) adopt those protocols for all their patients.

Recent Developments

The Return of Open Networks and the Rise of Tiering

New forms of health care delivery have emerged, including preferred provider organisations (PPOs), point-of-service (POS) plans, and "concierge care." PPOs involve a broad network of providers, who agree to accept discounted FFS payments in exchange for participating in the network. POS programmess generally require consumers to select a primary care gatekeeper, yet allow them to use out-of-plan providers for services in exchange for a higher co-payment. Some physicians who seek to avoid managed care entirely have begun concierge practices, where they provide personalized care, including house calls to patients willing and able to pay out of pocket for health care costs. The price of these options vary, with consumers facing greater out-of-pocket costs if they select less restrictive options. Health care financing has also moved toward a tiered system of payment. As the prior paragraph states, consumers pay less if they select a restricted managed care plan, or use an in-network provider than if they opt for a less restrictive plan or use an out-of-network provider.

The Road Forward

There has been considerable ferment in the health care financing and delivery markets in the last three decades. Such "creative destruction" is one of the benefits of a competitive market. Because no single arrangement is likely to satisfy everyone, diversity of financing and delivery options helps ensure that consumer welfare is maximised. Finally, competition is a process; as one commentator noted, "the superiority of open markets ... lies in the fact that the optimum outcome cannot be predicted."

Payment for Performance

In health care, payment has generally not been directly tied to the quality of the services that are provided. Numerous commentators have argued that payment for performance (P4P) should be more widely used. The Institute of Medicine (IOM) recently recommended that financing and delivery systems should "[a]lign financial incentives with the implementation of care processes based on best practices and the achievement of better patient outcomes. A prominent trade association of health plans similarly advocates using "payment incentives that reward quality care." An open letter in a prominent health policy journal similarly argued that strong financial incentives were necessary to motivate providers to improve quality. Other commentators suggest that "quality-incentive programmes should be viewed as part of a broader strategy of promoting health care quality through measuring and reporting performance, providing technical assistance and evidence-based guidelines, and, increasingly, giving consumers incentives to select higher-quality providers and manage their own health." Public and private payors are experimenting with P4P. Panelists noted that some providers have resisted P4P and tiering programmes, and refused to provide information regarding the quality of care they provide. Other panelists noted that providers are concerned about the reliability and validity of P4P measures, and the fact that payors are requiring them to invest in expensive equipment without providing additional funds or evidence that such investments are cost-justified.

Quality

Quality is an extremely important multi-dimensional attribute of health care. Many health services researchers and providers focus on whether the care that is provided is evidence-based. Economists typically view quality as a component of non-price competition. The IOM defines quality as "the degree to which health services for individuals and populations increase the likelihood of desired health outcomes and are consistent with current professional knowledge." The Agency for Healthcare Research and Quality (AHRQ) defines quality health care as "doing the right thing at the right time in the right way for the right person and having the best result possible." Regulators and most academic commentators have historically employed a three-part framework (structure, process, and outcome) to assess quality of care. Some consumers may focus on how long they must wait for an appointment, and how they are treated when they arrive at the provider's office. Depending on which of these attributes is emphasized and the particular condition being evaluated, it is possible for the same care to be simultaneously deemed high quality and low quality. Several commentators and panelists suggested that many health care providers and health services researchers view quality as effectively binary: a provider is either delivering high quality care to a particular patient or he is not doing so. This paradigm treats the resources of the individual consumer as immaterial to the determination of whether the care is of acceptable quality. Conversely, economists and legal scholars sometimes treat quality as an attribute that can be traded-off against price and other attributes of health care. Controversy can result from these differing conceptions of quality; in one Hearing session, panelists hotly disagreed over the appropriateness of conducting a cost-benefit analysis of improvements in quality.

Commentators and panelists agreed that health care quality actually encompasses many distinct factors, and the delivery system must perform well on each factor if it is to provide high quality care. These factors include whether the medical diagnosis is correct, whether the "right" treatment is selected (with the "right" treatment varying, depending on the underlying diagnosis and patient preferences and resources), whether the treatment is performed in a technically competent manner, whether service quality is adequate, and whether patients are able to access the care they desire without undue travel and inconvenience. Whether cutting edge technology and treatments are available is a component of health care quality, but it is not the only consideration. Information is necessary for consumers to make decisions about the care they will receive, and determine whether they are receiving the type of care they prefer and can afford. Competition has an important role to play in ensuring that consumers receive high quality care, and informing consumers of the costs and benefits of selecting a particular provider or treatment. Competition law promotes quality by encouraging consumer empowerment through information disclosure, and preventing market participants from engaging in anticompetitive conduct. At the same time, competition law provides considerable flexibility to market participants to act collectively to improve quality of care.

Health Care Quality

In recent decades, technology, pharmaceuticals, and know-how have substantially improved how care is delivered and the prospects for recovery. American markets for innovation in pharmaceuticals and medical devices are second to none. The miracle of modern medicine has become almost commonplace. Americans reap the benefits of new and improved drugs, cheaper generic drugs, treatments with less pain and fewer side effects, and treatments offered in a manner and location consumers desire. At its best, American health care is *the* best in the world. Commentators and panelists agree that providers are committed to delivering high quality care, that the vast majority of consumers are getting the care they need, and that there have been recent improvements in quality of care. There is, however, still significant room for further improvement. A 1998 literature review noted that there are large gaps between the care people should receive and the care they do receive. This is true for all three types of care—preventive, acute, and chronic—whether one goes for a check-up, a sore throat, or diabetic care. It is true whether one looks at overuse or underuse. It is true in different types of health care facilities and for different types of health insurance. It is true for all age groups, from children to the elderly. And it is true whether one is looking at the whole country or a single city . . . A simple average of the findings of the preventive care studies shows that about 50 percent of people received recommended care. An average of 70 percent. . . received recommended acute care, and 30 percent received contraindicated acute care. For chronic conditions, 60 percent received recommended care and 20 percent received contraindicated care.

Commentators and panelists stated that more recent studies have reached similar conclusions. In particular, commentators and panelists noted that treatment patterns vary significantly; procedures of known value are omitted; and treatments that are unnecessary and inefficacious are performed. Moreover, commentators and panelists noted that considerable sums are spent annually on services whose value is questionable or non-existent. As one commentator stated, "quality problems . . . abound in American medicine. The majority of these problems are not rare, unpredictable, or inevitable concomitants of the delivery of complex, modern health care. Rather, they are frighteningly common, often predictable, and frequently preventable." Commentators and panelists noted that medical treatments can injure consumers. The IOM estimated that medical errors during inpatient hospitalisation caused between 44,000 and 98,000 deaths per year - making medical errors the eighth leading cause of death in the United States. According to the IOM, every year medical errors in the hospital kill more people than motor vehicle accidents, breast cancer, and AIDS - without even counting the consequences of medical errors and low quality care in the outpatient setting. To be sure, these problems are not unique to American health care.

Commentators and panelists agreed that "in American health care, geography is destiny. Both the amounts and kinds of care provided to residents of the United States are highly dependent on two factors: the capacity of the local health care system (which influences how much care is provided) and the practice style of local physicians (which determines what kind of care is provided)." The cost of care varies as well: in the lowest quintile of regional spending, it costs an average of $3,922 per Medicare enrollee per year to provide care, while in the highest quintile of regional spending it costs $6,304 to provide care. One panelist noted that providers deliver more services in high-cost areas, but the additional services generally do not correspond to higher use of evidence-based protocols or better outcomes. For example, one study found 56 percent of the patients in the lowest spending region and 50 percent of patients in the highest spending region received optimal treatment for a heart attack. Similar patterns were observed for the provision of preventative care. One study indicates that there is an inverse relationship between Medicare spending per beneficiary and quality of care, and higher spending actually purchases lower quality care. To summarize, health care quality could be improved. The next section considers the beneficial role of competition in accomplishing this objective.

Competition and Quality

The relationship between competition and health care quality has not been studied as extensively as the relationship between competition and health care cost. One panelist reviewed the available studies and concluded that "the best evidence thus far is that quality is higher where we would think markets would be more competitive." More studies have been done regarding the impact of consumer information on quality. Information regarding quality allows consumers to make their own determinations of how best to balance those attributes that are important to them, obtain value for their money, and drive improvements throughout the system. If consumers are poorly informed about quality, providers may offer an inefficiently low level of quality. Not all consumers must be well-informed for the market to deliver an efficient level of quality. All that is required is that a sufficient number of consumers be well-informed about prices and quality levels of different sellers. These informed consumers can help drive the market to a competitive outcome. Consumers will use such information to select health plans, providers, and treatments that accord with their preferences if the information is presented in a usable fashion. Publicly available "report cards" can motivate providers to address quality deficiencies, even when it unclear whether consumers are relying on such information. Although competition can play an important role in enhancing quality of care, there are informational and payment barriers to effective competition. The next section turns to these matters.

Barriers to Improving Quality

Informational Barriers to Improving Quality

In many markets, consumers have ready access to reliable information with which to assess the quality of the goods and services they intend to purchase. Such information allows consumers to define and exercise their preferences along the dimensions of health care quality that are important to them. Information regarding quality is useful to consumers, providers, payors, and state and federal agencies. Unfortunately, in health care, such information is often difficult to obtain and is not necessarily reliable. Panelists discussed a variety of public and private sector initiatives for increasing the availability of information regarding quality. CMS has joined with hospitals and the Quality Improvement Organisations (QIOs) in Maryland, New York, and Arizona to design a group of pilot tests for publicly reporting hospital performance measures. There is also a voluntary public-private programme for reporting the same measures involving hospitals in every state. In addition, the Medicare Prescription Drug, Improvement, and Modernisation Act of 2003 provides that hospitals that report the requested data of quality will receive a full market basket update in hospital payments during 2005-2007, and hospitals that do not will have their payments reduced by 0.4 percent.

CMS has successfully used public reporting of quality information to improve dialysis care. Since public reporting began in 1996, the number of patients receiving inadequate dialysis or experiencing anemia declined substantially. CMS is currently using similar strategies for disseminating quality information regarding home health care and long term care providers. Similarly, in 1989, New York state began making provider-specific outcomes for cardiac surgery (including coronary artery bypass grafts (CABG)) publicly available. By 1992, one study found risk-adjusted mortality had dropped 41 percent statewide, giving New York the lowest risk-adjusted mortality. Studies show the mortality rate has continued to fall. Pennsylvania experienced similar improvements when it began collecting and publishing risk-adjusted report cards. Several other states provide either volume information for specific conditions or quality ratings based on clinical quality measures.

The National Committee for Quality Assurance (NCQA) also developed the Health Plan Employer Data and Information Set (HEDIS) to help assess health plans. HEDIS uses more than 50 measures of provider and plan performance in areas such as patient satisfaction, childhood immunisation, and mammography screening rates. HEDIS scores have been shown to affect employee plan choice. A number of other private initiatives seek to make similar quality-related information available to employers, health plans, and the general public. Additionally, AHRQ issues a national report on the state of the quality of care being provided.

Although information on quality is becoming more available, the benefits and costs of information-driven strategies are disputed. Panelists stated that consumers will use report cards if they are designed appropriately and the quality measures are sufficiently salient. One panelist noted report cards have not had the desired effects because "consumers are not aware of the quality problems that have been observed in health care," and that performance reports "have not really been designed to help people make choices." On the other hand, one study found that employers did not use data on quality to determine which health plans they should offer to their employees, and another noted that the use of performance measures for evaluating PPOs, which account for a growing share of the delivery market, is controversial. Several panelists noted that the usefulness of information disclosure depends on the target audience and the desired objectives. Different information and disclosure strategies may be preferable, depending on whether the goal is to "inform policy makers," "monitor progress over time," "provide some benchmarks for the future, identify some areas for improvement. . . [or] serve as a catalyst for action, both in improving quality and improving the quality of the measures and the data themselves." Panelists also noted that the disclosure of information to the public can "encourage professionals to recognize and fix deficiencies in health-care quality through a kind of self-regulatory behaviour." A variety of other concerns were also expressed about report cards and information disclosure strategies. One panelist stated that providers believe payors intend to use the results to lower payments to providers instead of improve quality.

Commentators and panelists identified concerns about the clinical validity and generalizability of particular measures, the time-lag between treatment and the generation of the report card, the way in which results are risk-adjusted, and how consumers will react to the information. Commentators and panelists also stated that information disclosure may discourage providers from treating high-risk patients, and result in "gaming" of the system.

One panelist suggested that providers would be more willing to collect information if that information was not made available to the public. Several panelists indicated that providers believe information disclosure will confuse consumers and cause malpractice litigation. In general, the Agencies encourage information dissemination, because it allows consumers to make better informed decisions. In addition, commentators and panelists agreed that providers are less likely to modify their behaviour if information is not publicly available. Public reporting of quality measures can be a powerful incentive for providers to improve. It is important, however, to keep the costs, limitations, and potential adverse consequences of information disclosure strategies in mind. To be useful, an information disclosure strategy must balance cost-effectiveness, clinical validity, and consumer saliency. Finally, information technology (IT) is an important part of making information available to consumers, providers, and other interested parties. Panelists and commentators agreed that the health care marketplace does not employ information technology extensively or effectively.Prescriptions and physician orders are frequently hand-written. Records are often maintained in hard copy and scattered among multiple locations. Few providers use e-mail to communicate with consumers. Public and private entities have worked to develop and introduce electronic medical records and computerized physician order entry, but commentators and panelists agreed that much remains to be done.

2. Payment Barriers to Improving Quality

Commentators and panelists agreed that there is not a "business case for quality" in health care because payment arrangements are rarely tied to the quality of the services that are provided. The IOM observed that "current [compensation] methods provide little financial reward for improvements in the quality of health care delivery, and may even inadvertently pose barriers to innovation." The Medicare Payment Advisory Commission more bluntly noted that "at times providers are paid even more when quality is worse, such as when the complications occur as the result of error." These problems are not theoretical. After Duke University Hospital created an integrated programme to treat congestive heart failure, consumers were healthier - but the hospital lost money because of the resulting decline in admissions and the absence of complications. In Utah, ten hospitals had a similar experience after implementing practice guidelines for pneumonia treatment. One panelist noted that current payment systems for end of life care create an economic disincentive for providers who deliver "key elements of chronic care."

Commentators noted that existing payment arrangements may paradoxically make providers financially worse off if they are better at delivering health care than their competitors. Such payment arrangements are economically perverse: no rational system of compensation rewards an agent (the provider) for making a principal (the consumer) worse off.

At any given level of payment, commentators and panelists agreed that providers are less likely to improve quality of care if they suffer financially when doing so.

Commentators and panelists also agreed that investments in quality improvement are similarly likely to be inadequate when costs are front-loaded, and benefits are deferred - particularly if the providers and payors incurring these costs will not capture the benefits. Public and private payors and providers are seeking to address these problems by creating direct economic incentives for the delivery of high-quality care (pay for performance or P4P). CMS recently introduced a demonstration project that pays modest financial incentives for hospitals that score in the top 20 percent and modest financial disincentives for hospitals that score in the bottom 20 percent on specified measures of quality for five conditions. There are significant statutory impediments to broader use of such incentives by CMS in the Medicare programme.

Employers and private plans are also experimenting pay for performance and other strategies to reward providers that adopt processes that are believed to improve quality. The Pacific Business Group on Health has been using incentive-based performance targets for eight years in its contracts with HMOs. HMOs that fail to meet targets for patient satisfaction and various clinical benchmarks (including prenatal care, mammography, pap smears, childhood immunisations, and cesarean section) forfeit two percent of their fees. The Leapfrog Group, a coalition of 145 private and public organisations, is using its purchasing power to encourage hospitals to adopt computerized physician order entry (CPOE), referrals to high volume hospitals for certain procedures, and staffing intensive care units (ICUs) with intensivists. Although more than a thousand hospitals are participating in Leapfrog, one survey showed that only six percent of hospitals had fully implemented CPOE, 57 percent had fully implemented ICU physician staffing, and most hospitals were meeting one to two of the six targets for referrals to high volume hospitals for selected procedures. A number of large health plans and hospital networks are also experimenting with such arrangements. Tiering can also be employed to link financial incentives to quality of care. Commentators and panelists agreed that, to date, P4P has had limited impact on the health care marketplace.

Quality, Competition and Competition Law

"Enhancing quality" has long been the invariant excuse of providers who engage in anticompetitive conduct. As Chairman Robert Pitofsky noted when testifying before Congress on behalf of the Commission, quality-of-care arguments "have been advanced to support, among other things, broad restraints on almost any form of price competition, policies that inhibited the development of managed care organisations, and concerted refusals to deal with providers or organisations that represented a competitive threat to physicians." There are almost always more narrowly tailored means of achieving the same quality improvements without employing the anticompetitive means selected by self-interested providers.

Some commentators and panelists stated that antitrust law impedes providers' efforts to improve quality. Providers actually have considerable flexibility to act collectively to improve quality of care. Through their professional societies and other groups, health care professionals can jointly provide information and express opinions to health plans and the general public.Physicians, for example, may collectively explain to a health plan and the general public why they think a particular policy or practice is medically unsound and may present medical or scientific data to support their views. Finally, the Agencies have *never* brought a case based solely on providers' collective advocacy with a health plan on an issue involving patient care. Competition law also enhances quality in ways that are not widely appreciated. When providers engage in anticompetitive conduct they can undermine the quality of care actually received by the population as a whole. Lower prices can actually contribute to higher quality; as several commentators noted, "when costs are high, people who cannot afford something find substitutes or do without. The higher the cost of health insurance, the more people are uninsured. The higher the cost of pharmaceuticals, the more people skip doses or do not fill their prescriptions."

Stated differently, when anticompetitive conduct increases prices, it makes it more difficult for many Americans to obtain needed care. Estimates of the price elasticity of health insurance vary, but many small employers do not offer health insurance at all because it is too expensive. When employers offer health insurance, price increases can result in limitations on coverage, employees refusing to sign up for insurance, and employers dropping coverage.Numerous studies establish that the lack of health insurance is associated with deleterious consequences, including increased mortality. Thus, anticompetitive conduct that raises prices, even if it is done in the name of improving "quality," is likely to have a systemic adverse effect on the quality of care actually provided to the population as a whole. In a competitive market, consumers consider various dimensions of quality and price. Competition law exists to promote and enhance consumer choice along all of these dimensions.

Provider complaints about the antitrust laws miss the point of those laws. As one commentator noted:

> [T]he antitrust laws are concerned with maximising the long-term welfare of consumers, but this is not inconsistent with the interests of efficient providers. The providers who are most efficient and offer the best-quality service at reasonable

> prices will attract patients in a competitive environment protected by the antitrust laws. The providers whose methods fall behind the times and who rely on the protection of concerted action to maintain their position may lose ground. But that is precisely what one should expect in our free enterprise system.

In an efficient market, consumer preferences specify the targets at which providers aim. When providers engage in anticompetitive conduct, they frustrate this process. By ensuring a competitive marketplace and transparency of information, competition law and policy allows such demands to be satisfied, and prevents self-interested provider groups from preempting "the working of the market by deciding for itself that customers do not need that which they demand."

Basics of Competition Law

Federal competition law stems from a series of federal statutes, principally the Sherman Act, the Clayton Act, and the Federal Trade Commission Act.

The Sherman Act prohibits unilateral and collective conduct that poses unacceptable dangers to competition. Section 1 of the Sherman Act declares unlawful "every contract, combination ... or conspiracy, in restraint of trade," while Section 2 of the Sherman Act prohibits "monopolisation" and "attempted monopolisation." Courts reviewing Section 1 cases generally focus on whether the allegedly conspiring parties reach agreement, and whether that agreement was unreasonably restrictive. By contrast, courts reviewing Section 2 cases generally examine whether the defendant created or maintained a monopoly through wrongful or exclusionary means. The Clayton Act prohibits mergers and acquisitions where the effect "may be substantially to lessen competition, or to tend to create a monopoly." The Clayton Act thus reaches incipient threats to competition that might escape the Sherman Act's reach. Under related legislation, parties to proposed mergers that exceed statutory thresholds are required to notify the federal antitrust agencies of their plans and afford the government a limited opportunity to investigate before the transaction is executed.

Finally, the Federal Trade Commission Act provides that "unfair methods of competition in or affecting commerce, and unfair or deceptive acts or practices in or affecting commerce are ... unlawful." The Supreme Court found this provision provides the FTC with the authority to attack conduct constituting a Sherman Act violation. The FTC Act provides no criminal penalties and is limited to equitable remedies. Depending upon the specifics of a case, the Commission enforces the FTC Act either administratively or through the courts. Advisory opinions are available for parties interested in prospective guidance as to the strictures of the FTC Act. The Division offers business review letters that perform much the same function for the statutes that the Department of Justice enforces.

The Agencies are the primary antitrust enforcement authorities, although state attorneys general and private parties can also bring suit. For example, both the Division and private parties may sue to enforce the civil provisions of the Sherman Act, which authorize treble damages and broad equitable relief. By contrast, only the Division may enforce the criminal provisions of the Sherman Act. Moreover, the federal laws assign each Agency responsibility to enforce various antitrust laws. Thus, both Agencies can pursue violations of the Clayton Act, but only the Commission may enforce the FTC Act.

Because most of the antitrust challenges to health care practices focus on allegedly anticompetitive agreements, an abbreviated analysis of the standards for assessing such claims is warranted. In reviewing such claims, "the development of horizontal restraints jurisprudence suggests an analytic framework that proceeds by several identifiable analytical steps." Some conduct - such as naked agreements among competitors to fix prices or allocate markets - is viewed as "inherently suspect owing to its likely tendency to suppress competition." Such arrangements "always or almost always tend to raise prices or reduce outputs." Such conduct merits summary condemnation to prevent long, expensive investigations and litigation over conduct that is almost certain to cause harm to consumers. Most of the time, however, "conduct cannot be adjudged illegal without an analysis of its market context to determine whether those engaged in the conduct or restraint are likely to have sufficient power to harm consumers." Depending on the case, the necessary analysis can be sweeping or relatively constrained. As several panelists noted, antitrust investigations are factually intensive, and "antitrust cases have to be done one at a time."

INTRODUCTION TO COMPETITION LAW AND HEALTH LAW

As background to the succeeding chapters, this chapter summarizes the basics of competition law and offers a brief history of the application of competition law to health care markets. This chapter also provides an abbreviated overview of several specific forms of regulation that affect the structure and performance of the health care marketplace.

Application of Competition Law to Health Care

Courts, lawmakers, and commentators once believed that health care markets should not be subject to competition. Thus, it was widely understood that there was a "learned professions" exception to the antitrust laws; government enforcers or private parties only rarely pursued anticompetitive conduct in health care. The existence of this exemption remained an open issue until 1975 when the Supreme Court explicitly determined that the antitrust laws apply to "learned professions." One year later, the Supreme Court held that the alleged acts of a hospital were "sufficient to establish" a "substantial effect" on interstate commerce under the Sherman Act.

In *Arizona v. Maricopa County Medical Society,* the Supreme Court emphasized that the antitrust laws applied fully to the health care marketplace. The Court found that an agreement among physicians to set maximum prices charged to policyholders was *aper se* violation of the Sherman Act.

For almost three decades, the Agencies have continued to enforce the competition laws by initiating investigations, filing and litigating complaints, filing amicus briefs in private litigation, and writing advisory opinions and business review letters for the health care industry. The Agencies took an additional step in the application of competition law and policy to health care by issuing the joint *Department of Justice and Federal Trade Commission Statements of Antitrust Enforcement Policy in Health Care (Health Care Statements)* in 1993. The Agencies designed the *Health Care Statements* "to advise the health care community in a time of tremendous change, and to address . . . the problem of uncertainty concerning the Agencies' enforcement policy."

In response to comments and changes in the health care marketplace the Agencies expanded the *Health Care Statements* in 1994 and amplified them again in 1996. The *Health Care Statements* currently specify a range of circumstances that will not provoke enforcement actions (also known as "safety zones") for hospital mergers, hospital and physician joint ventures, physicians' provision of information to purchasers, multi-provider networks, and joint purchasing arrangements among health care providers.

The *Health Care Statements* also provide a number of examples applying antitrust analytical principles to a particular set of health-care related organisational arrangements. The Agencies also offer prospective guidance relating to health care through advisory opinions and business review letters. Finally, the Agencies have jointly filed amicus briefs in a number of cases, including a recent brief filed in the Sixth Circuit, explaining the Agencies' analysis of how the state action doctrine should be applied to the conduct of subordinate state entities, such as public hospitals.

Commission Health Care Related Activities

The Commission has long challenged barriers to competition in health care markets to foster innovative and more efficient means of delivering and financing health care. In the last several years, the Commission has made special efforts to protect competition in pharmaceutical markets, given rapidly rising drug expenditures that are causing great concerns among patients, employers, and government officials. The Commission has been especially active in investigating and challenging conduct that excludes or unduly delays generic competition from pharmaceutical markets. It has also reached important settlement agreements in mergers in the pharmaceutical markets, and successfully argued in an amicus brief that improper pharmaceutical filings before the Food and Drug Administration are not immune from antitrust review.

The Commission also issued a recent, comprehensive study on generic drug competition. This study recommended legislative changes to the statutory framework governing generic drug entry to mitigate the possibility of abuse of this framework. Most of these recommendations were enacted by the Medicare Prescription Drug and Improvement Act of 2003. Since the 1970s, the Commission has had an active law enforcement programme targeting anticompetitive practices among physicians and other health care professionals. The types of conduct within the health care professions that have been subject to Commission challenge over the decades include agreements on price and price-related terms, agreements to obstruct the entry of innovative forms of health care financing and delivery, and restraints on advertising and other forms of solicitation.

Since 2002, the Commission has entered into 17 consent agreements with physicians, their organisations, or their non-physician consultants and agents, settling charges that the respondents have engaged in unfair methods of competition - primarily involving joint contracting with payors and other forms of price-fixing. Additionally, Commission staff are currently evaluating the effects of consummated hospital mergers in several cities. The Commission will announce the results of these retrospective studies after determining whether the mergers in question were harmful to consumers. One case arising out of this investigation is currently in administrative litigation.

Division Health Care Related Activities

During the last three years, the Division has pursued formal investigations across the full range of healthcare products and services. In addition to the matters on which it has taken formal enforcement or advisory action, the Division has examined, or is investigating, mergers and conduct of managed care organisations, including the review of four major mergers of health plans. In one of these matters, the Division publicly set forth the reasoning that led it to clear the formation of the nation's largest health plan. The Division has examined both vertical contracting arrangements involving health plans and providers as well as allegations of horizontal agreements among plans.

Additionally, the Division has or is investigating mergers and conduct of providers (both physicians and hospitals), including allegations of horizontal agreements. These investigations, while not resulting in challenges, have included criminal inquiries into the conduct of managed care plans, hospitals, and physicians.

The Division's civil conduct investigations have encompassed hospital conduct, blood products, and retrospective examinations of a hospital joint operating agreement and a multi-hospital joint selling venture, the latter of which implemented mechanisms intended to achieve clinical integration without formal merger. The Division's formal merger investigations have encompassed hospital mergers, senior assisted living facilities, and diagnostic imaging service providers. Finally, the Division has actively provided counsel to the Administration on health care policy matters.

The Division has taken several public enforcement actions, including a merger challenge involving critical care monitors and orthopedic equipment, litigation resulting in a consent decree against the Federation of Physicians and Dentists, a case brought against the dominant producer of prefabricated artificial teeth in the United States, and a consent decree requiring dissolution of a physician organisation of over 1000 members.Additionally, the Division has issued favourable business review letters to two groups requesting guidance regarding fee surveys.

Private Litigation

The majority of antitrust challenges to health care activities arise in private litigation. One study showed that the Agencies brought only six percent of the antitrust challenges to health care practices involving quality of care from 1985 to 1999. Most private antitrust challenges are not successful: the same study found that plaintiffs won favourable opinions only 14 percent of the time; 67 percent of the judicial opinions favoured defendants, and the remaining 19 percent favoured neither party. The most common private antitrust healthcare litigation claims involved staff privileges and exclusive contracting cases.

Health Law Overview

The states and the federal government extensively regulate health care. Many of these regulations are described in greater detail, *infra*. This section provides a basic introduction to several important provisions that are important to understand the health care marketplace.

Anti-Kickback

The Medicare and Medicaid Anti-Kickback Statute (42 U.S.C. §1320a-7b(b)) broadly criminalizes the solicitation or receipt of remuneration in connection with items or services for which payment is made under Medicare or Medicaid. There are statutory exceptions for discounts, payments pursuant to a bona fide employment relationship, group purchasing organisations, waiver of coinsurance obligations, and risk-sharing agreements of managed care organisations. There are also administrative regulations creating specific safe harbors and advisory opinions covering a number of other arrangements. Those who violate the anti-kickback statute are subject to criminal and civil penalties and/or exclusion from participation in the Medicare and Medicaid programmes. The anti-kickback statute has had an important effect on the structure of the health care marketplace.

Self-Referral Amendments

The Self-Referral Amendments (42 U.S.C. §1395nn) prohibit physicians from referring Medicare and Medicaid patients to ancillary providers in which they or their family members hold a financial interest and prohibit service providers from billing for services performed as a result of such referrals. The Self-Referral Amendments apply to certain designated health services. A financial interest includes an ownership interest or a compensation arrangement (the latter includes both the giving and receiving of compensation). There are certain defined situations in which a physician is permitted to receive payment for the referral of a Medicare or Medicaid patient to an entity in which he or she has a direct or indirect financial interest, including when the physician has an ownership interest in a whole hospital. The Self-Referral Amendments create a strict liability offense, with violation punishable by programme exclusion and substantial civil penalties. Like the anti-kickback statute, the Self-Referral Amendments have had an important effect on the structure of the health care marketplace.

Medical Malpractice

Medical malpractice litigation is governed by state tort law. To prevail in a medical malpractice claim, the plaintiff must prove that the provider-defendant owed a duty of care to the plaintiff, that the provider-defendant breached this duty by failing to adhere to the standard of care expected, and that this breach of duty caused an injury (with associated damages) to the plaintiff. Malpractice litigation seeks to compensate negligently injured consumers, deter unsafe practices, and achieve corrective justice. Numerous panelists and commentators stated that the medical malpractice system is in the midst of a crisis. The American Medical Association (AMA) has declared a malpractice crisis in twenty states, claiming that important health care services are in short supply. Complete consideration of this issue lies beyond the scope of this Report, but it significantly affects the health care marketplace.

EMTALA

The Emergency Medical Treatment and Labor Act (42 U.S.C. §1395dd) requires hospitals that receive Medicare funding and have an emergency department (ED) to provide an appropriate medical screening examination to any individual who comes to the ED and requests one. Stabilizing treatment must be provided to individuals with an emergency medical condition. Violations are punishable with civil penalties, programme exclusion, and private lawsuits brought against individual hospitals. Like the anti-kickback and Self-Referral Amendments, EMTALA has had an important effect on the health care marketplace.

Obligational Norms

Many members of the public view health care as a "special" good, not subject to normal market forces, with significant obligational norms to provide necessary care without regard to ability to pay. Similarly, risk-based premiums for health insurance are perceived by many as inconsistent with obligational norms and fundamental fairness, because those with the highest anticipated medical bills will pay the highest premiums. A wide array of regulatory interventions, ranging from EMTALA and mandated benefits to community rating and guaranteed issue, reflect these norms.

Commentators have extensively analysed the application of competition and antitrust law to health care. In general, these commentators have concluded that increased competition has empowered consumers, lowered prices, increased quality, and made health care more accessible. The Agencies have long held that standard antitrust analysis and doctrines apply to health care markets. With rare exceptions, the antitrust laws are rules of general applicability, and they govern health care markets in largely the same way that they govern other markets. To be sure, as noted previously, health care is extensively regulated. The optimal balance between competition and regulation is an enduring issue. Just over thirty years ago, the Senate Judiciary Committee, Subcommittee on Antitrust and Monopoly held six days of hearings on Competition in the Health Services Market. Senator Philip A. Hart opened the hearings with the following prescient observations:

> Over the years, health care service has been treated pretty much as a "natural monopoly." It has been assumed that a community could support only so many hospitals; that providers just naturally control supply and demand. And there may be validity to such ideas. But, in this area, as in many others which have long been thought of as "natural monopolies," today questions are being raised as to just how pervasive the monopolisation must be. Isn't it just possible, some are asking, that turning competition loose, at least in some sections, may not only lower the costs of health care but improve its quality? . . . [W]e hope to develop some suggestions as to areas where restrictions on trade could be replaced with competition to the benefit of the health and pocketbooks of consumers.

In the intervening thirty years, it has become clear that health care is not a natural monopoly, and that competition has an important role to play in ensuring that consumers can obtain the care they desire at a price they are willing to pay. The Agencies help maintain competition in the health care financing and delivery markets, and ensure that market participants can compete to satisfy consumer demand.

THE FINANCIAL STING — PAYING MORE FOR LESS

Bob Ingram of La Canada, California lives on a fixed income and is disabled due to cancer. In May 1999, Ingram received a troubling letter from his wife's HMO, Prudential. "Your monthly premium will be increased by 21%," the letter read.

"Who can afford $8,000 per year in medical care with all the other expenses associated with going on with life?" asks Ingram. "When you don't have any more money coming in, and they are raising their premiums at this pace, it's mind boggling. You are cornered." Managed care was premised on lower costs, but these promises now ring hollow. Americans now face double digit premium increases and rising co-payments and deductibles to insure themselves. The nation's largest non-profit HMO, Kaiser Permanente, raised its premiums in 1999 by 12% for state employees and as much as 50% for individuals. Humana raised premiums 11% to 12% for big employers and 15% to 16% for smaller groups. The Federal Employees Health Benefits Plan, which covers all federal employees and is an important market barometer, had a 10.2% increase in premiums in 1999. Didn't HMOs contend that they could deliver quality medical care at reasonable cost? If patients have not been getting quality care, where did all the money go? The final insult of corporate medicine is that it has been a financial swindle. In Medicare, for instance, HMOs in 1998 began dropping senior patients in many counties because the companies' reimbursements were not high enough. In 1999, the HMOs told the federal government what they are now telling every other purchaser of health care — you will have to pay more for less. Aetna testified before Congress in March 1999 that "If the current reimbursement structure is not adjusted, more Medicare-Choice organisations are likely to withdraw from areas served and beneficiaries enrolled in the remaining plans will likely experience premium increases or reduced benefits."

In response, Congressman Pete Stark, ranking Democrat on the House Ways and Means Committee said, "As I've already described, we currently pay Medicare HMOs more than we should. We pay the plans more for the people they enroll than we would have paid if those people had stayed in Medicare fee-for-service. To rephrase that, the taxpayers would actually save money if we abolished the Medicare-Choice programme today."

What incensed Congressman Stark most was that the HMO industry wanted a programme of "premium support" that would require every Medicare recipient to choose an insurance program, with higher premiums charged to beneficiaries who pick traditional fee-for-service Medicare. The proposal is essentially a full employment act for HMOs because, as Stark says, "it is just a way to raise premiums on seniors and the disabled to force them into bare-bones, no-frills HMOs that will offer no extra benefits...If plans say they cannot offer extra benefits at a time when we are overpaying them, they certainly won't be able to do so if Medicare were to actually start saving money by paying them more accurately for the people they enroll. And, if plans cannot offer extra premiums, who would want to join a system that rationed their choices and services?"

United States Senator Jay Rockefeller, Representative John Dingell and Representative Jim McDermott — who sat on the Bipartisan Commission On The Future of Health Care — agree with Stark and provide a larger context for American HMO medicine's failure: "We never seriously looked at the experience of foreign countries. All the other major industrialized nations (except Australia) have older populations than the United States, yet they are able to insure all their citizens, with reasonably good quality care, for about 30 to 50% less of their Gross National Product than we spend.

The Congressmen quote a 1999 report of the National Academy of Social Insurance: "The United States...has the unfortunate distinction of spending relatively more per capita for the elderly while providing them with less comprehensive coverage with generally higher out-of-pocket costs." What happened to the claims that corporate-managed services can deliver quality medical care at reasonable cost? Where does all that money go? One promise of managed care was that health maintenance and managed care organisations have a built-in incentive to keep patients well by providing preventive health care. Some of the best programmes do try to keep patients well by providing alternative health care options and frequent screening rather than wait for serious problems to develop. Alternative medicine or health club membership can help Americans stay healthy. It is when patients become ill that the deficiencies of HMO medicine are clear. As evidenced by the stories and statistics in this book, corporate medicine has failed to exhibit caution in treating illnesses in the most timely and least expensive manner. The promise of managed care of long-term cost reduction has proven ephemeral. Some 20 to 30% of our premiums now pays for overhead — to enrich industry executives and an army of bureaucrats — even as nurses are fired to save money and doctors are required to spend as much time with industry paperwork and obstacles as they do on treating patients. Numerous studies from sources such as the California Medical Association and the *New England Journal of Medicine* have documented the increasing money from our premiums going to the corporate bottom line. Indeed, in "managed care" speak, any money spent on patient care is a "medical loss." This speaks volumes about the goal of corporate medicine — not to lose money on patient care.

In addition to rising deductibles and co-payments, the insurance industry is shifting every health care cost it can back on patients. Many Blue Cross patients, for example, recently found themselves forced into a bind: take much higher deductible policies or pay rate increases of up to 58%. Many *insured* Americans find simple surgery can cost them thousands of dollars in out-of-pocket expenses. Orthopedic surgery typically requires serious rehabilitation and physical therapy. Any shoulder or knee surgery, for instance, can require months of physical therapy to avoid further surgery. Many managed care policies, even the more expensive preferred provider plans, typically place strict time limits (say thirty days) on any physical therapy. So a patient can face the choice of more surgery or paying for physical therapy out of pocket. This absurd approach may lead to some patients having more surgery (presumably covered by insurance) to avoid paying for rehabilitation costs out of pocket.

These are only some of the effects as insurers becoming increasingly monopolistic, with growing power to rapidly escalate premiums in order to squeeze out more profit. Another symptom of this power is the narrowing freedom that HMO doctors are allowed to exercise in writing prescriptions. Physicians are charted like race horses based on the costs of the prescriptions they write, sometimes regardless of the wellness or age of the patient population they serve. Patients are forced to pay for less effective over-the-counter medications rather than receive prescription drugs at a cost to the HMO. Some HMOs exclude the most effective prescription remedies in favour of cheaper, older drugs. Because of rising costs, employers, in fact, are scaling back retiree health coverage for pharmaceuticals. Mental health coverage, too, has been squeezed with strict limits on therapy, and, perversely, because it is cheaper, a desire to shun therapy and instead prescribe medication.

And what of the uninsured? The promise by the architects of for-profit managed care was lower medical costs, thus expanded access for Americans without insurance. In 1988, prior to the national recession, managed care had 29% of the health care market and there were 36 million uninsured or 17% of the public. Now with a booming economy and near full employment, managed care controls 61% of the market and there are 43.4 million uninsured or 19% of the public. The ranks of the uninsured are growing by close to a million Americans per year. Seventy-five percent of the uninsured are gainfully employed. In this system, where the public increasingly pays more money for less coverage, who wins?

The Robber Barons of Health Care

HMO executives have piled up truly extraordinary sums of money for themselves. Even if we accept the industry's argument that executive compensation is a result of stunning new management techniques and the elimination of inefficiencies, the money in the executives' pockets formerly was spent on health care. Does HMO executive compensation really reach the levels of the robber barons of old? Former U.S. Healthcare CEO Leonard Abramson, now on the board of Aetna, made over $990 million when U.S. Healthcare was acquired by Aetna. The merger was valued at nine billion dollars. This means over 10% of the companies' value ended up in his bank account. Remember the story of Betty Hale, forced to raise $30,000, one dollar at a time, to provide the downpayment on the breast cancer treatment that saved her life. Even so, she came out of it still owing $184,000. The money pocketed by Abramson could have paid for *four thousand* of these kinds of treatments!

Mr. Abramson may be the most striking example of appropriating our health care premium dollars but too many HMO executives live like sultans. Ironically, while Wiggins topped the 1997 list for pay, his company crumbled that year — recording consistent losses after computer problems caused it to lose track of billing records and medical costs. Too often, executive compensation and a company's performance bear little relation to one another.

Dr. Malik Hasan, recently forced from his position as CEO of Foundation Health, is a walking illustration of how to get rich from the current health care system. A neurologist by training, he quickly left his medical roots after he began a small Colorado-based HMO. Dr. Hasan embarked on a ferocious merger and acquisition binge that resulted in Foundation Health becoming one of the largest managed care organisations in the nation. Hasan had the dubious distinction of making the *Forbes* magazine list of "overpaid" executives during the nineties, the group of corporate chieftains who "made out far better than shareholders since 1993." Even as Foundation's stock plummeted, his annual salary was in the millions. No blushing violet, Hasan stated, "we are being innovative, and we are helping to solve some very difficult and knotty problems. If we are successful, then I think we deserve not only this, but more." Those "customers" of Foundation Health who were denied or delayed treatment to help amass the millions in pay and options may not agree with Dr. Hasan's definition of success. Dr. Hasan was also quoted about the problems of the uninsured and underinsured: "We are not in the business of social redistribution." Hasan claimed it is the not-for-profit companies that "have a responsibility they have not fulfilled" and they should be doing more to care for the indigent. Dr. Hasan also made no bones about profiting from the conservative's favourite health care idea, medical savings accounts. "We [for-profit managed care companies] would make out like bandits, but as a physician I have a serious concern about fragmenting the insurance pool...We are going into [MSAs] because these things are going to be a gold mine, let there be no doubt. They are a scam and we will get our share of that scam." It's a dirty job, but someone has to profit.

What is so exceptional about overpaid CEOs? Every industry has them. One answer is that HMO executives like those listed above are among the most highly paid CEOs in the country. The *Crystal Report on Executive Compensation* found HMO chiefs' compensation outpacing their CEO counterparts in other industries by a factor of two to three. After analysing the pay packages of 1,568 CEOs in thirty-one industries and accounting for company size and stock performance, the study found that HMO executives topped the list, trailed by CEOs of drug manufacturers and biotech companies, brokerages and computer companies. But does their pay, large though it is, really burden the system? The answer is yes. One study found that the stock-related wealth of just the top twenty-three managed care executives would provide:

— health insurance for six million people, *or*
— health coverage for 14% of the nation's uninsured or alternatively 18% of California's entire population.

In 1996, analyst Don DeMoro added the estimated stock wealth of HMO executives ($6.9 billion) to the combined five-year profits of twelve select managed care companies ($8.8 billion) to the approximate amount of merger and acquisition activity in health care from 1992 to 1996 ($134 billion). This combined amount would provide comprehensive health insurance for 130 million Americans. That's over half of the population currently insured. In a democracy, how amounts of money this large are spent on a public commodity like health care ought to be the subject of major civic debate. Instead, the fate of precious health care resources is decided behind closed doors in corporate boardrooms.

As Dr. Eli Ginsburg notes, current government health care expenditures in the United States approximate 7% of the Gross Domestic Product. This is the same percentage that Britain spends to provide health care for all its citizens. When one adds all the money employers and individuals pay in an American system that still leaves more than 17% of the public uninsured, it is clear the profits currently skimmed from the system prevent more comprehensive approaches. Even one of the pioneers of HMO medicine has come to agree with this conclusion. Dr. Robert Gumbiner, the founder of Fountain Valley, California-based FHP, made a lot of money through his company, but insists that his primary concern as a doctor was his patients and providing access to affordable health care. His staff model HMO grew out of a physicians' group to service patients under the original HMO theory that all services would be under one roof at a reduced cost. In discussions in 1997, Gumbiner stated that he believes modern HMOs, that own no medical resources but simply contract with doctors and hospitals to provide care, should be regulated like public utilities. He charged HMOs had become too easily manipulated by the greed of corporate officers and Wall Street, causing patients to suffer.

"The present orientation towards greed is a national catastrophe, as far as I can see," said Gumbiner. "The feeling is, it's okay to be greedy and it's okay to exploit your fellow man just to line your pockets. To me, there is something wrong with that...Quality and investment return are antithetical, because in order to generate short-term profits, the company cannot put money into research and development, new long-range concepts, management training, and all the things that will build a long-term successful organisation. So people who strictly have investors' return as their motive are not interested in long-term corporate guarantees." Why did Gumbiner have a change of heart about the system he helped to found? Gumbiner contends that following a bout with cancer he was forced from the helm of his company by venture capitalists who conspired to defraud FHP shareholders of over $200 million during the 1997 sale of FHP to PacifiCare. He alleges numerous violations of the federal Securities and Exchange Act. The allegations, made in conjunction with the lawsuit filed in a Los Angeles federal court, paint a troubling portrait of a handful of insiders seizing control of a health maintenance organisation and strip-mining it of its value to long-term shareholders, patients, medical personnel and the public. According to the allegations, "dressing up" FHP for sale involved the dismantling of its medical infrastructure and forward-thinking medical programmes in order to reduce overhead costs and make the HMO attractive to any new suitor. Gumbiner revealed that corporate officers not only fired one-third of FHP's doctors to make the company attractive to potential buyers, but went so far as to round up all the potted plants at the HMO and put them in a dark room to die rather than paying for a housekeeper to water them. The FHP-PacifiCare consolidation was only one in a series of HMO mega-mergers in the 1990s demonstrating that money, not patient care, is the driving motivation of the new medical regime.

As managed care companies squeezed more profit from premium dollars, the HMOs piled up so much money that by the end of 1994, Margo Vignola, a Solomon Brother's analyst, estimated the nine biggest publicly traded HMOs were sitting on $9.5 billion in cash. Using this money from premium payments, they soon began to buy up smaller competitors. "Our problem is what to do with the money that comes in, not whether we have enough cash," said Alan Bond, the treasurer of Health Systems International.

At that point, the HMO had $475 million in cash in the bank with $15 million pouring in every month. A spending spree soon ensued in the managed care industry, not one that would help patients, but one designed simply to make more money for management and shareholders. Eighteen of the largest for-profit HMOs and managed care companies have now been reduced to six gigantic companies: Aetna, CIGNA, United Healthcare, Foundation Health Systems, PacifiCare and Wellpoint Health. (Kaiser, a non-profit, is the only other HMO in this company.) As Robert Hoehn, director of stock research at Solomon Brothers, recently noted, "The industry in the 21st Century will comprise a few diverse large companies who have pushed out the niche players." While this now seems inevitable, effective anti-trust action could prevent this course. Unfortunately, the Clinton Administration has been asleep at the switch, failing to break up any major HMO merger to date. Acquisition and consolidation in the managed care industry is what led to inflated executive compensation packages at the top. Like many industry consolidations, mergers in health care limited choice and drove down services, as the cost of the acquisition had to be absorbed. Health care consolidation has meant riches for the few and downsizing for the rest of us. As the California Medical Association noted during the merger of PacifiCare and FHP, numerous studies indicated few new efficiencies in managed care mergers but merely fewer dominant companies that increased prices and cut services.

For a while this game of musical chairs was possible because Wall Street investors kept bidding up the shares of certain managed care companies. These companies with inflated share prices gobbled up each other as well as community hospitals and non-profits. But then the zero sum financial nature of managed care became increasingly clear, as many companies reported losses and one time "write-offs." Kaiser Permanente lost $270 million in 1997. Stock prices for corporations like Columbia/HCA and Oxford Health collapsed, the latter plummeting by 70%. An August 1998 merger between Humana and United Healthcare to create the largest managed care organisation failed when stock prices took a nose dive. Foundation Health Systems, Mr. Hasan's source of wealth, saw its stock drop from thirty-two to five by February 1999. This slump in stock prices may not be short-lived. As Joseph Nocera, editor at large of *Fortune* magazine, observed: "Consider the root cause of the swoon in health stocks. After years of cutting costs with impunity, managed care companies are forced — in no small part as a reaction to intense criticism from doctors and patients — to pay more for treatment." But industry analysts do not discount the role that mismanagement, waste and greed in the race to grow at all costs has had on corporate stability.

Looming Bailout

Merger mania has begun to increase prices and restrict choice for patients. The glory days for HMO stocks seem past, now that all the low-hanging fruit has been picked. New profits can be squeezed only from doctors' fees, patient services and raising premiums. In fact, in the spring of 1999, some of the largest companies, like PacifiCare and Aetna, posted significant profits from their premium increases and decision to dump more costly Medicare patients. The depressed stock prices of some of the weaker companies left them as easy pickings for the largest companies. Where will all these mergers lead? A peculiar possibility is the creation of health care organisations that are "too big to fail." This will be the ultimate perversity, the taxpayer being called upon to subsidize the avarice of top managed care management. This is not just a far-fetched worse case scenario; it already occurred in New York when the taxpayers provided funds for Empire Health in 1993. In New Jersey, an HMO called HIP recently had to be taken over by the state. In 1999, the state of California seized a physician-run medical management company, MedPartners, that served 1.3 million patients. On paper, the company itself had no employees, or assets regulated by the state, only the value of its parent corporation, which said it had no obligation to debtors. A similar failure of San Diego-based FPA Medical Management Corporation left doctors on the hook for tens of millions of dollars in bills for services already rendered.

Sound familiar? Is it like the Savings & Loan bailout, which cost taxpayers up to $400 billion to rescue after quick-buck operators of these deregulated operations went down in fraud and flames? As Michael Schrage, a consultant at MIT noted, "HMO networks will not go bust lending money to aspiring Texas mall moguls or Arizona real-estate developers. The issue here is not bad loans and rising interest rates, it's balancing promised business performance with promised quality and quantity of care. That is becoming ever harder to do." In addition, many HMOs are heavily leveraged and an economic downturn or prolonged stock slump could lead to further bankruptcies. State and federal regulators have often been slow to look at the impact of mergers on the health care of patients, even as the twin goals of market return and quality medical care now appear mutually exclusive. HMOs cut back to maintain profits in a number of ways — fewer referrals, less treatment, less caution with regard to patient health. Moreover, accountability also suffers. Why worry about fines or sanctions if you hope to sell your company before the lethargic regulatory environment catches you?

The corporate logic favouring monopoly is pushing towards a few giant health care concerns that manage the care for most Americans. To get a snapshot of where the country stands in this spiraling trend toward monopoly, one need go no farther than Aetna's proposed buyout of Prudential's health care business. Despite the slump in profits, or perhaps, in some cases, propelled by it, consolidation continues:

— Aetna currently provides care for one in every twelve Americans; after the merger it will be close to one in eleven.

— 38% of the HMO market in New Jersey will be controlled by the company and over 50% in other small markets. "Our concern is that when a doctor's practice is more than 20% with any carrier, it becomes almost impossible to say something is unacceptable," said Dr. Greg Bernica of the Harris County Medical Society in Texas.

— Aetna will control 39% of the market in Philadelphia, 30% in Atlanta and 33% in Orlando, Florida.

As competition disappears, one impact of this concentration will be increased premiums. Professor Glenn Melnick, a specialist in health care finance at USC, stated the relationship like this: "When the number of competitors goes down, the level of price competition also goes down." One can also expect less generous benefit packages and lower levels of basic care for the money. As health care expert Charles Blankersteen noted, "Choice in the marketplace is rapidly diminishing, customer service and value are less than spectacular. Who bears the cost of these acquisitions? My bet is the people who buy the services." In other words, you and I do.

Aetna has yet to integrate the last two companies it absorbed, New York Life in 1998 and U.S. Healthcare in 1996. Three years after the merger, doctors and patients of

U.S. Healthcare continue to have problems with service. Perhaps what is most telling about Aetna's ongoing consolidation are the patients' and doctors' views. According to a 1998 survey in *U.S. News and World Report*, Aetna ranks last among insurers in customer satisfaction in nine states (Connecticut, Georgia, Illinois, Maryland, Massachusetts, New Hampshire, New York, Texas and Virginia). In five of these states, Aetna is among the biggest three insurers. In California, Aetna was ranked dead last in an opinion survey of doctors conducted by the Pacific Business Group on Health Negotiating Alliance. One consequence of being the biggest company is that patients and physicians have little leverage to maintain the quality of care. The stranglehold such a company has over physicians is profound. Aetna has employed gag orders on doctors to prevent informed choice by patients. The company has been charged by regulators in New York and Florida with the failure to comply with state laws. Four hundred doctors in Texas, 600 in San Jose, California and over 500 in Southern California have walked out recently due to Aetna's cut-rate reimbursements and contract clauses.

Aetna has tried to foist upon doctors the requirement that they either sign onto all Aetna's plans or they not be allowed to do business with any of its plans. With this "all or nothing" approach, the insurer tries to force physicians who accept any form of insurance from the company to accept all forms. As Dr. Howard Weiner, head of a 1,200 member physicians association noted, "This policy in essence drives the market to all HMO care." Concerned about Aetna bullying doctors in this way, lawmakers in Texas, Illinois and Rhode Island are considering bans on such all-or-nothing clauses. The North Dakota Senate has passed a prohibition and the Nevada Insurance Commissioner has stopped the practice. Physician concerns about only participating in plans that allow them to meet both their ethical and financial goals, since some plans have higher reimbursements and fewer restrictions on treatment options and referrals, have fallen on deaf ears at leviathan Aetna. Why should Aetna listen? It has expanded because of its callousness towards physicians' concerns — which has enabled the company to cut costs and conserve cash for purchases.

Financial Failure of the HM-itos

One of the newest problems is that HMOs have foisted onto physician-run medical groups responsibility and risk they are incapable of handling. The State of California takeover of the financially bereft, physician-run medical group, MedPartners, dramatizes the newest vice spawned by HMO medicine — physicians practicing insurance without a license. When HMO bureaucrats with MBAs started to tell MDs what to do, the physicians' political establishment responded. It created another mid-level bureaucracy run by physicians, called the medical group, to manage risk, like an insurer does. Like the HMO, the medical group receives a "capitated" rate, only from insurers instead of employers. Like the HMO, the financial incentive for the medical group means the less done for patients, the more it makes. The arrangement has won the medical groups the designation "HM-itos" among insiders. The medical group system was once touted by some as a middle ground for managed care because doctors purportedly had control again. But as the financial collapse of MedPartners and FPA show, these groups can be financially unsound.

William Sage, who teaches health policy at Columbia University Law School, says, "The entities that are most vulnerable tend to be contractors that have been the most aggressive in terms of growing their companies." In fact, HMOs have paid to physicians capitated rates that are so low that it would be virtually impossible to take care of patients' real medical needs. In one case, doctors are reported to have received as little as $6 dollars per patient per month from an HMO to manage all their needs. Because there are so many doctors and so few HMOs, doctors have little leverage in their negotiations. If a medical group receives an HMO contract, among so much competition for them, the group has probably agreed to take whatever reduced-rate the HMO will pay. When an HM-ito like FPA or MedPartners fails, it is the patient who pays with disruption to the continuity of care. "It's high anxiety," said Edward J. Gold, an oncologist who had patients with the failed HIP Health Plan of New Jersey. "Many patients are afraid. They don't know what's going to happen."

The *Los Angeles Times* reports that the parents of twins recovering from premature delivery were told by their HMO that the children must be moved crosstown from one hospital to another because of the bankruptcy of FPA. FPA's failure forced the primary-care doctor to switch medical groups. That led the doctor to affiliate with a new hospital.

"The Raffertys did not want to break the close ties they had developed with the medical staff at the hospital, especially when it would mean putting Paige and Hannah in the care of people less familiar with the twins' histories," reported Stuart Silverstein and Davan Maharaj. "But the HMO told the Raffertys that they might be responsible for all future hospital-related costs — expenses that wound up totaling hundreds of thousands of dollars — if they refused to allow the babies to be transferred."

Moreover, so much money is spent on bureaucracies to manage risk that the dollars actually spent on patient care has dwindled to a pittance. The irony is that the mounting administrative costs of insuring, not caring, for patients is what is driving health premiums up. If the HMO takes 20% right off the top for its own business costs, overhead and profit, what does a medical group take? What is paid to the medical group may be reported as a "medical loss" by the HMO (i.e., dollars spent on treatment), but the medical group must then take from this remaining money its administrative costs. These include a burgeoning number of "medical directors" whose job is to say "no" to other physicians who request care. They track and compare the costs of doctors' prescriptions and treatments in fancy bar graphs. Then with remaining dollars the medical group must buy reinsurance, so-called stop-loss insurance, to cover the cost of any catastrophic care that, for instance, a cancer patient may need. In perhaps the biggest financial scam in the system, medical groups are said to even buy stop-loss insurance from the same HMO that passed them the full-risk capitated rate in the first place. So the HMO profits twice.

The Political Muscle of the Insurance Industry

Where does an increasing amount of HMO cash go? Unfortunately, to Capitol Hill lobbyists and Madison Avenue spin-doctors. Growing monopolies mean more than rising premiums, constraining doctors, cutting care, and foisting costs onto patients. It also translates into political power. The insurance industry has added hundreds of millions in profits during the rise of managed care and is spending significant sums of this money to preserve its dominion. It defeated the Clinton health plan through its misleading "Harry and Louise" ads and millions in lobbying dollars. It is laughable that the centerpiece of the insurance industry advertising campaign concerned the inability to consult with your family physician under the Clinton plan. The proposal may have been overly complex and bureaucratic, but the industry has since limited coverage, choice and access to specialists in a manner never envisioned by the Administration. Today, "Harry and Louise" would be cast as a woman unable to get a mammogram annually and a man unable to schedule a cardiogram — the victims of corporate bureaucrats, not government employees. The Patient Protection Bill introduced by Senator Edward Kennedy and Congressman John Dingle and endorsed by President Clinton is the best opportunity to reduce the industry's power over health care decisions. It would, among other things, hold the insurance companies legally accountable for denying medically necessary care. In March of 1999, the Business Roundtable launched yet another round of multi-million dollar television advertising against the plan during the NCAA basketball championships. The ads compare reforms allowing patients the right to sue their HMO with playing roulette and refer callers to the HMO industry's 1-800 hotline to send a message to Congress. Another multi-million dollar ad campaign is underway at this writing in the summer of 1999. Republicans, who by and large oppose liability for the insurance industry, read the 1998 polls and did offer cosmetic reforms. The party made no real attempts to pass even these reforms, preferring to defeat the Democratic proposals and attempt to increase the strength of anti-reform forces in the 1998 election.

The message was not lost on the insurance industry in 1998. The industry certainly responded with its wallets. Direct contributions to candidates from the health insurers doubled between 1994 and 1998. Certain favourites like Republican Congresswoman Anne Northrup reportedly received more than 10% of their total contributions from the industry in return for leading the fight against increased patient protection. The industry was also active in so-called issue ads. The American Association of Health Plans spent a considerable sum against the Senate challenge of Democrat

John Edwards in North Carolina who campaigned heavily on behalf of patients rights. The ads vilified trial lawyers and stated Americans would lose their health care if patient protection measures passed. The voters thought otherwise, and Edwards won a narrow victory.

Frank Pallone, a six-term New Jersey representative, also learned the dangers of opposing the insurance industry. A front group, Americans for Job Security, spent over $1.2 million trying to defeat Pallone after his aggressive promotion of the Patient Protection Bill. Over one million of the organisation's $7 million advertising campaign against pro-HMO reform Democrats was reported as a grant from the insurance industry. Pallone still won handily.

One estimate of total industry spending during the first six months in 1998 for direct lobbying to defeat managed care reform topped off at $60 million. This averaged $112,000 per member of Congress. This outrageous sum of money, of course from patients' premiums, does not include direct candidate contributions nor $11 million in "feel good" advertising. This figure dwarfs the estimated $40 million spent by the tobacco industry to defeat federal anti-smoking legislation. The chief spokesman of the Texas Medical Association questioned why the health plans do not spend premium dollars on medical care: "If this were about patient care, they would shift the money into patient care aspects, therefore dissipating some of the consumer insurrection. What this is really about is control and power. It speaks volumes about their intent."

The industry has already announced its plans to spend millions of dollars in New Hampshire and Iowa to affect the outcome of the presidential primaries in 2000 and will no doubt spend tens of millions in 1999 and 2000 in the renewed effort to prevent federal and state regulation. The industry, with allies such as the Chamber of Commerce, is intent on maintaining a stranglehold on the health care of the American public.

Corporate for-profit medicine has as its core principle interests inimical to any American who is seriously ill or injured. Unfortunately, over the course of time, this is the fate of almost all of us. The message from the industry to its captive customers is clear. Profits will be protected at all costs. Unless the public rallies to support meaningful reform, the industry will continue to curtail medical care to maintain profits. One of the founders of the HMO concept was Paul Ellwood, MD. He recently noted, "For those of us who devoted our lives to reshaping the health system trying to make it better for patients, the thing (managed care) has been a profound disappointment.

Climbing Out of the Spiral: Health Care Professionals and Others Fight Back

This trend of consolidation and its deleterious effects are becoming clear to many. Princeton health care expert Uwe Reinhardt echoed Wall Street analyst Hoehn, noting, "The health system is stumbling toward a bilateral monopoly of insurance companies and provider groups in every market. If only one provider is left in a community, it will send the bill to the consumer by raising premiums. The government can then say, 'You have converted health care into a public utility, we need to regulate you.' " Indeed, if there is to be a role for profit-making monopoly health care in our future, it will have to be regulated much like an electrical utility. A reasonable amount of administrative overhead and return on investment would be allowed in return for strict compliance with public standards. This, of course, will be derided by some as socialized medicine, but it merely acknowledges that the market must be regulated in health care. As Professor Reinhardt notes, "If these plans keep buying each other up, there is no longer competition, because executives of the plans can regulate everything they want in one golf game."

How did we get to this point in the monopoly spiral? Large employers clearly were looking to control their health care costs. The strategic underpinning and promises of managed care were promoted by corporate think tanks. Miracles were promised from market-based solutions. Employers signed on. Without full public debate about the wisdom of managed care, Americans now find themselves pushed into HMOs by their employers. Sixty percent of Americans insured through their employers have no choice in health plans and another 20% have only a choice between two plans. In reaction to a system designed for profiteering that has been squeezed on many fronts, doctors and nurses have rebelled, increasingly unionizing to confront the HMO bosses. The historic approval of a doctor's union by the American Medical Association in June 1999 is instructive. Americans should realise that the concerns of doctors should be their own. What stands in the way of a few corrective regulations? One unfortunate answer is the employers who pay for much of the insurance. The mantra the insurance industry and the Washington, D.C. trade associations employ today is, "Regulation will lead to increased costs and less coverage." This statement by some corporate employers that increased regulation will drive up costs indicates the often shredded nature of the social compact between employers and employees. It is emblematic of the times that most employers side with for-profit insurers rather than their own employees in health care decisions. If top executives were forced to endure the vagaries of managed care then perhaps we would see real change. Many in top management, however, enjoy gold-plated fee-for-service policies — the kind that used to be available to everyone. Allen Meyerson of the *New York Times* noted, "Many of the nation's largest corporations — including Atlantic Richfield, Charles Schwab, RJR Nabisco, SBC Communications, Gannett — are leading more by precept than example."

The increasing complaints of employees have led some companies to join their employees in the search for increased quality health care. Some employers are indeed rethinking their allegiance to these insurance companies. Bruce Bradley, director of managed care plans for General Motors, noted recently he was, "very concerned that the health care industry is moving away from local delivery and HMOs are becoming more like insurance companies." It behooves our large employers to look at quality of care not just cost in seeking medical care. The managed care industry is merely an expensive middleman. Companies can begin to contract directly with non-profit hospitals or organisations of doctors.

In the meantime, corporate medicine continues to exact its financial toll not only on resources for patient care, but on academic medicine and charity care as well. Two March 1999 studies published in the *Journal of the American Medical Association* found that in regions where managed care saturation is greatest, physicians are less likely to give the poor free care and academic institutions are less likely to spend their money on scientific research. Ten thousand physicians and 2,000 faculty members were surveyed. Dr. David Blumenthal, director of the Institute for Health Policy at Massachusetts General Hospital and author of the medical-school study, said the results show that where HMO medicine predominates, the ability to work toward "the common good" evaporates. America's great teaching hospitals and medical school physicians are the envy of the world. The current regime of financing has, however, helped strangle research and left elite physicians with ponderous paperwork fighting insurance companies to pay for required treatment in their clinical practices. The medical school mission is not merely to make money, but to train physicians and conduct cutting-edge research, as well as treating the poor. Urban medical schools frequently end up treating complicated cases from publicly supported hospitals. This is not a recipe for making money. Financial gain should not be the mission of our advanced medical institutions. Academic medicine should not be merely advanced clinics forcing physicians to see patients in a rushed manner. This is the case in many medical schools today.

If our society is going to commit less in public dollars to academic medical centers because we are training fewer doctors, then the money must come from somewhere. One solution could be a dedicated tax on HMO profits to support regional academic medical centers. The health care system benefits greatly from these institutions. As Dr. Harvey Shapiro notes, "Some type of per head tax on HMO revenues should be assessed to develop a trust fund for academics and other functions such as independent oversight, technology assessment, and standards-setting boards." Medical schools often treat patients with the most difficult and complex diseases or conditions. In addition, any effort to transfer risk to physicians via capitation or any other schemes will naturally hurt physicians who employ their skills treating the sickest patients. According to a recent report by the Commonwealth Fund, medical schools and their clinics make a unique contribution to communities by delivering highly specialized care. For instance, although academic medical centers are only 2% of all community hospitals, they are 47% of trauma units, 46% of burn units, and 31% of HIV/AIDS units. Managed care plans push patients away from academic medical centers, because of higher costs. This deprives these centers of clinical revenues which helped subsidize complex patient care and the disproportionate number of Medicaid and charity cases these hospitals take as referrals.

Teaching hospitals provide nearly 40% of the nation's charity care. How have the financial pressures impacted academic medicine's mission? "It's a total crisis, a complete crisis," said Neil Rudenstine, the president of Harvard in April 1999. "I think anybody who would call it less than that would really just not know what's going on. I'm not quite sure what the cumulative deficit of our four or five closely related hospitals is, but it's certainly well over $100 million, and we haven't even finished the year yet." UCSF Stanford Health Care lost $50 million in 1999 and expects to layoff 2,000 of its 12,000-person staff. Peter Van Etten, the center's chief executive, said, "I have to say the services we will provide can't be of the same quality that we would provide with 2,000 more people." Academic hospital downsizing has also sparked an unprecedented push towards discouraging doctoring. The nation has more than 700,000 physicians. As a result, the federal government has, for the first time, agreed to pay hospitals around the nation hundreds of million of dollars *not* to train doctors. Hospitals that limit their number of residents receive more federal funds. The idea is to give hospitals an incentive to save money.

Academic medicine has also been hurt by declines in medical research despite increased funding of the National Institute of Health in the nineties. The Administration, though, is proposing only a 2% increase in FY 2000. The United States now spends less per capita on medical research than England, Denmark and France. Research is too often conducted by pharmaceutical companies hoping to cash in with exorbitant prices on lifestyle enhancing drugs. Unchecked corporate medicine will certainly facilitate this transition. .

3

Children and Health Care Services

AN INTERSECTORAL RESPONSE TO CHILDREN WITH COMPLEX HEALTH CARE NEEDS

The purpose of this paper is to stimulate debate on how to define and enact public responsibility to children with complex health care needs and their families. National and provincial policies define accountability at a macro level and are not intended to be prescriptive at the micro level. Indeed, principals, teachers and service providers would be critical of the involvement of policy makers in micro-management. Yet, decision-makers focus on the shortcomings of existing policy and not on the shortcomings of management. For example, the Children and Youth Home Care Network has called for "governments at all levels to assign higher priority to developing coherent policies for children with special needs and families, particularly in the home and community". Spalding and colleagues reported that service integration and coordination would not improve until there are "fundamental changes at the broader system level.... There is no urgent need for policy to 'catch up' with reality. Rather there is a need for principals, teachers and service providers to develop programmes that support policies. This study details a case study of an evidence-based programme that provides the critical link between the policy and good practice. This programme involves Community Care Access Centres, schools and Saint Elizabeth Health Care, a complex-care nursing provider. The case study illustrates how public responsibility has been successfully enacted at a local level within existing policies for children with complex health care needs.

Statement of the Problem

Children with complex health care needs have a profound impact on families and on the educational system. Parents believe that their employment status is affected and we know that they have difficulty in finding childcare . The impact on the educational system, which has increased over time and is projected to further increase, is driven by three factors. First, the Canadian Charter of Rights and Freedoms ensures that every child with either a mental or physical disability has the right to access educational services. Compliance with the Canadian Charter, the Education Act and regulations in Ontario requires each school to provide all special needs children with a free and appropriate public education in the least restrictive setting. School principals are required to ensure that an Individual Education Plan (IEP) is developed for each child who has been identified as "exceptional". Second, children who previously would not have lived are now surviving, and through technology are being cared for in the community . Finally, Canadians want greater choice and input into planned services, and want to be confident that these services are efficient, effective and of high quality . To meet the needs of the growing number of children, educators must work with individuals from sectors outside of education . Sectors are distinct public service systems such as health and education. Intersectoral policies define the shared responsibilities for the welfare and well-being of a distinct population group. In Ontario, the intersectoral mechanism for children who require health support services is Policy/Programme Memorandum Number 81 (PPM 81). PPM 81 outlines the responsibilities of three sectors: Education, Health, and Community and Social Services [Ontario Ministry of Education, 1984 #5]. The Ministry of Education is responsible for the administration of oral medication, physical assistance, physio/occupational therapy, and speech and language services. The Ministry of Health and Long Term Care is responsible for the injection of medication, catheterization, manual expression of bladder/stoma, postural drainage/ suctioning, tube feeding, and speech therapy. The Ministry of Community and Social Services is responsible for all services in children's residential care/treatment facilities.

The Ontario intersectoral mechanism for children with complex health care needs has been implemented in Toronto by five Metro Toronto Community Care Access Centres (CCACs) through the School Health Support Services (SHSS) programme. These CCACs are responsible for co-ordinating in-home and in-school community-based health services for children and youth, in particular the provision of an extensive care for children with complex long-term disabilities. They see to the planning, co-ordinating, and delivering of professional SHSS programmes support. The SHSS programme enables children with health support needs to attend school with their peers . In addition, the SHSS provides health related education, teaching, and consultation services to staff and parents in the school setting. At the local service level, the Metro Toronto CCACs contract through a "Request For Proposal" process, with three health care agencies to provide nursing care in the school-based programme. The three agencies are 1) Saint Elizabeth Health Care (SEHC), 2) Victorian Order of Nurses (VON) Toronto-York Region, and 3) Comcare Health Services Limited.

Saint Elizabeth Health Care (SEHC) is one of the health care providers invited by CCACs to respond to principals' request to deliver health care in an educational setting.

The organization has been an active participant in the delivery of paediatric programmes since 1908. In its early years, nurses provided mostly prenatal and paediatric care, making their way to homes on foot or by streetcar. Essentially a Toronto-based nursing organization until 1994, SEHC now provides a full range of health care and services through 17 Service Delivery Centres from Windsor to Cornwall, and as far north as Thunder Bay. It contracts with over half of the CCACs in Ontario and delivers more than two million visits to over 150,000 individuals and families annually.

SEHC's multidisciplinary team of more than 2,500 staff includes Registered Nurses and Registered Practical Nurses, Occupational Therapists, Physiotherapists, Personal and Home Support Workers, Nutritionists, Speech Language Pathologists, Social Workers, Chaplains and Mental Health Professionals. With well-established programmes in the areas of nursing, personal support and rehabilitation, SEHC was one of the first home health care organizations in Ontario to be awarded an accreditation by the Canadian Council on Health Services Accreditation. The clinical areas of excellence are Child and Family, Long-Term Care and Gerontology, Mental Health, Palliative Care and Rehabilitation. Some examples of SEHC's specialty services include Advanced Wound Care, Home Infusion, Diabetes Management, Crisis Intervention and Maternal Newborn Care. In addition to expanding geographically and broadening its scope of services, SEHC is now offering professional consulting services nationally and internationally, and leveraging technology to provide quality, accessible care. To help SEHC successfully lead community health care into the 21st century, the Saint Elizabeth Health Care Foundation was incorporated in 1997 to raise charitable support for the enhancement and expansion of superlative home health care services in Canada. The Foundation supports advances in health care research and technologies, continuing education and technical training, and the ongoing development and implementation of innovative programmes and services. As a testament to SEHC's very caring values and commitment to making a valuable contribution to the communities it serves, the Foundation has sponsored the printing and distribution of two illustrated, easy-to-follow guides by Harry van Bommel, respectively titled *Caring for Loved Ones at Home* and *Family Hospice Care: Pre-planning & Care Guide*. Over 100,000 copies of each book have been distributed, free-of-charge, to hospitals, hospices, home care organizations and individuals to help family caregivers effectively manage and respond to the home care needs of their loved ones.

Child and Family Programme

Saint Elizabeth Health Care provides high quality family-centred care based on its commitment to research of child and family issues and the implementation of research/evidence-based practice. The Child and Family Programme is guided by principles of family-centred care and the organization's values respect the unique needs and expectations of its client families. Professionals with advanced knowledge in community-based child and family care co-ordinate SEHC's comprehensive interdisciplinary team approach. This approach ensures seamless consultation and collaboration with experts to mobilize a range of resources and health care options to meet unique child and family needs. SEHC's teams recognize the diversity of the community environment and adapt care according to the social, ethical and economic factors that affect families. The Child and Family Programme includes the following services:

— Perinatal Services

— Complex Care School Nursing Services

— Complex Care Home Nursing Services
— Acute Care Nursing Services

From birthing mothers to infants and adolescents, the Child and Family Programme promotes optimal health and wellbeing through health teaching, illness management and support to families in adjusting to ongoing health challenges. SEHC also provides health teaching to professionals and caregivers to support the wellbeing of children in their care.

SEHC's definition of health is guided by the World Health Organization's determinants of health and includes physical, intellectual and emotional/social dimensions. The philosophy of family-centred care is built on the cornerstones of collaboration, information sharing, encouragement and support. Staff respect the lifestyles, values, beliefs and culture of families and respond with accessible, flexible and empowering services. For example:

— SEHC supports families to participate in all decisions about care planning and delivery.
— SEHC respects the family's knowledge and expertise in caring for their child.
— SEHC builds on family strengths and foster independence.
— SEHC adapts interventions to meet the child and family's changing needs.
— SEHC customizes care strategies that support the child and family's unique response to health and illness.

The goal of SEHC's children's services is to promote the health maturation of the child within the context of the family/community. SEHC assists the child and family to achieve, maintain and promote optimal levels of health; facilitates rehabilitation and improvement of the child's ability to function; identifies threats to the child's health and well-being; and facilitates the management of health challenges.

Programme Features

Saint Elizabeth Health Care's paediatric nurses are educated and experienced in advanced paediatric nursing. They are additionally certified to provide specialized services for all age groups. These include:

- Provision of IV and TPN therapy
- Wound management
- Diabetic treatment and teaching
- Suctioning and chest percussion/postural drainage
- Tube feeding
- Irrigations
- Catheterization
- Chest tube care
- Ostomy care
- Ventilator care
- Chang Tracheotomy care
- Pain management
- Behavior management
- Central line care
- Cardio-respiratory care
- Psychosocial assessment and support
- Cast care

Practical Problems with Implementation of Policy/ Programme Memorandum Number 81

SEHC's Child and Family Team assessed the quality of

care received by children with complex health care needs. Several weaknesses were noted:

— Parents commented that they were not contacted prior to school enrolment.

— Continuity of care was compromised by nurse turnover.

— Parents wanted more frequent communication about school events.

— Communication among health care providers, the school and the CCAC was sub-optimal.

— The lack of coordination/integration with the school authorities undermined the quality and accountability of services.

— There were no clear guidelines regarding the service protocols.

— There were no standards for staff qualifications.

— There were limited opportunities for the providers to improve their skill set.

— Standardized monitoring of the care delivered in the school was limited.

— Performance appraisal of nurses was not conducted.

— Inadequate attention to problems reduced accountability.

— Limited advocacy services increased the costs for parents.

— The lack of daily leadership reduced the quality of partnership services.

CASE STUDY

Rationale and Description

In recent years, many public sector organizations have examined the subject of accountability. This has been initiated by extensive changes in the delivery of services and in the increasing use of partnering arrangements to deliver public programmes. To an increasing extent, there is some form of shared accountability. In our case study SEHC nurses, teachers, principals, three Ministries, the CCAC and the family shared the accountability. These partners could not afford to wait for the introduction of policies that require organizations share accountability. Instead, the partners introduced change voluntarily through an effective accountability framework that built on the Auditor General of Canada's five principles of effective accountability :

Clear roles and responsibilities – For all sectors in the accountability relationship, roles and responsibilities must be well understood and agreed upon.

Clear performance expectations – The health care objectives pursued and outcomes expected are to be explicit, understood and agreed upon.

Balanced expectations and capacities – Performance expectations must be clearly linked to and aligned with each sector's capacity to deliver.

Credible reporting – Credible and timely information must demonstrate what was achieved, and what was learned.

Reasonable review and adjustment – Fair and informed review and feedback on performance must be carried out by all sectors, achievements recognized, corrections made, and appropriate consequences for individuals was carried out.

Description of Protocol

The protocol developed by SEHC incorporated the 5 principles of shared accountability and was designed to address documented shortcomings in care delivery.

Clear Roles and Responsibilities

- Children are now admitted to the school programme before the first day of school. During the summer months, a Primary Nurse meets with the child and family in the home. A partnership is initiated with the family at this time. Effective collaborative planning is ensured at all times with the family, CCACs and the school staff.
- The CCACs assess the needs of the child or youth and their families and communicates that assessment to the nurse.
- If additional visits are required, then the CCAC is asked to approve payment.
- The Primary Nurse meets with the teacher before the start of school to discuss the child's educational, health and psychosocial goals. A collaborative planning process is initiated.
- SEHC's Manager of Child and Family Services meets with principals to clarify roles and responsibilities; telephones parents and arranges to have satisfaction surveys conducted. Professional relationships are developed and resources needed to support nursing activities are put in place.
- SEHC visits principals with CCAC Case Managers. Meetings may include nurses delivering services at the school.
- SEHC finds similar employment for the Primary Nurses during the summer months and has

documented that the current retention of these well-qualified nurses is very high.

- In schools where more than one nurses provides services, a team leader communicates with CCACs, principals and SEHC.
- There is improved partnership between SEHC Service Coordinators, school authorities and parents.
- A communication log is updated and sent home daily to the parents.
- Prior to the introduction of the communication log, nurses were phoning parents on an as needed basis to communicate issues such as need to replace equipment, requests for more feeding supplies, changes in health status etc. (Nurses were finding it difficult to make personal contact with parents during the workday, and so much communication was in the form of messages left on answering machines or brief phone exchange at times inconvenient for families and outside of work hours for nurses. In addition, many of the children in the programme were unstable, and nurses wanted to know how the child had slept or about seizure activity at night. For children receiving overnight nursing, this communication was in the form of a voicemail report from the night nurse to the school nurse. Some children were transported to school accompanied by a nurse, so nurse/parent contact happens at the beginning and end of the school day.)

Note, however, that a significant number of children were exceptions to the above generalizations. Some parents were sending notes to the nurse in the child's backpack. Educational assistants, teachers or intervenors would read these notes, however, and nurses often found them unhelpful for a variety of reasons.

The Communication Log was created to address this issue. It is clearly labelled and kept in a large envelope marked confidential. It travels daily in the child's backpack. It allows the nurse to communicate daily and to address a broad range of issues from the child's developmental successes to number and quantity of feeds. Parents can also respond and ask questions about their child's health. This daily communication allows the nurse to expand her care giving beyond the child to include parents or primary caregivers. Nurses and parents are exchanging journals, newspaper articles of interest and photographs. Nurses are reporting high satisfaction from the improved therapeutic relationship that includes parents.

Clear Performance Expectations

— Primary Nurses attend professional development activities arranged by the tertiary care hospital for children.

— Training such as g-tube feeding and deep suctioning are provided to Primary Nurses by the tertiary care hospital.

— Nurses are receiving training at tertiary hospitals specifically from care providers in the hospital who are providing care to these children so the training is customized to the unique needs of the child being admitted to the school programme. SEHC's relationship with the Hospital for Sick Children is such that the transition from hospital to community is smooth. Health care needs are not compromised as the child enters school.

— Regular meetings are held through the years on Professional Development days.

— In addition school nurses are attending meetings as a programme team 5 times per year mainly for clinical education and to discuss operational issues and challenges unique to school nursing. Significant transfer of knowledge occurs from expert school nurses to novices who are working within a politicized, unionized educational environment. Nurses learn about leadership and how to establish respectful relationships with multiple disciplines.

— There are standards for staff qualifications.

— Clear guidelines regarding the service protocols have been established.

— Skills in communication, roles and responsibilities in school politics are developed to enhance multidisciplinary engagement. Professional relationships are built with school personnel and teachers.

Balanced Expectations and Capacities

— SEHC meets with principals of all schools in late August to set expectations and how to work together.

— SEHC liaises with other sources of funding to streamline service delivery with the consent of the child and parents.

— To deliver quality care, SEHC offers extended hours of respite care for working parents, both before and after school.

Reasonable Review and Adjustment

— Periodic review meetings and a conflict resolution process are established for all stakeholders. SEHC's Manager of Child and Family Services conducts site visits, audits charts, and appraises the performance of all Primary Nurses on an annual basis. SEHC's Manager of Child and Family Services resolves minor issues directly; and is involved in problem resolution of more substantial issues with the CCAC.

— School personnel communicate minor problems directly through nurses to SEHC before reaching the CCACs and SEHC communicates with CCACs.

Credible Reporting

— SEHC visits schools and meets with principals, teachers and caregivers in the school.

— SEHC conducts performance appraisals with nurses.

— SEHC conducts site visits to ensure health and safety.

— SEHC audits client charts.

— Parental satisfaction is regularly monitored.

Clientele

From 1999 to 2002, SEHC provided school based complex health care service to 131 children. Of this number, 27% (36 children) were 5 years of age or less, 36% (47 children) were from 6 to 10 years of age, 23% (30 children) from 11 to 15 years, and the 16 to 20 years olds represented 14% (18 children). Females totalled 58 (44%) and males totalled 73 (56%). Analysis of the administrative data confirmed that these children had complex health care needs. Seventy-eight (78) diagnoses were identified for children served in the school health programme. The most frequent diagnoses were: 44 developmental delay (56%), 44 seizure disorder (56%), 26 cerebral palsy (33%), 10 asthma (13%), 10 feeding problem (13%), 9 diabetes (12%), and 8 quadriplegia children (10%). As large as 73 % of the total children served had multiple diagnoses, underlining the complex nature of the health care needs. The most frequent reasons for referral to the school programme were: G-tube feeding, chest physiotherapy, g-tube medication, suctioning, and tracheotomy care.

Methodology

The perceptions, attitudes and opinions of principals and complex care nurses caring for these children by SEHC were obtained through 1 to 1.5 hour key informant interviews at each school. The interviews were audio taped with the permission of the interviewees, which were later cross-checked with the notes taken during the interviews. Three team members used modified content analysis as a procedure to make valid inferences from text . One investigator reviewed the transcripts and notes from the interviews and identified themes. Another investigator independently examined the groupings of themes and made some revisions. The revised list then served as the foundation for another investigator to reanalyze the key informant interviews. A few new themes were identified and agreed to during this process.

Results

Themes identified through modified content analysis were grouped under three headings: Enablers, Outcomes, and Areas for Improvement.

Enablers

Four enablers identified by the principals and the Primary Nurses were four of the key components of the SEHC protocol: 1) ongoing support; 2) ongoing monitoring; 3) Communication; and 4) Professional development. The interviewed nurses recommended that all nurses and teachers caring for children with complex health care needs meet with their Supervisor prior to the start of school to discuss roles and responsibilities and ensure that environment/ resources support their activities. The nurses felt that this orientation was critical in fostering an awareness of the roles and responsibilities of individuals in each sector. In addition to these four components of the SEHC programme, the principals and nurses identified respect and CCAC resources as enablers. Primary Nurses felt that the principals respected their skill set. The principals felt that the nurses were respectful of the educational environment and participated in school functions. Finally, the resources provided by the CCAC (Time, Talent, Information and Supplies) were seen as enablers.

Outcomes

Four outcome-related themes were identified through the modified content analysis: 1) Increased quality of and longevity of life; 2) Increased access for children with complex health care needs; 3) Principals' satisfaction; and 4) Improved access to health care services by principals. According to the Primary Nurses and principals, after receiving medical and education services, the children have made improvement in their functional goals and maintained that improvement. For example, advanced gross motor skills and speech sound production were improved in some of the children. The Primary Nurses said they were highly satisfied with the support services they delivered which are family-centred and functionally oriented. Furthermore, changes in government policy have permitted the delivery of health services at schools that were formerly provided only in intensive care units in institutions.

Areas for Improvement

Two themes were identified as areas for improvement: 1) Increased awareness; and 2) funding or wage parity. The key informants expressed their concern over the limited awareness of other professionals and the public of the SHSS programme. The nurses indicated that they wanted other nurses, even within their own health care agency, to be aware that there are highly skilled nurses working in the educational sector. Finally, inadequate funding support was the last theme identified in the modified content analysis. These nurses have chosen this work because they view the work as a calling. However, there is a chronic shortage of skilled nurses willing to work with the children with complex health care needs . The nurses stated in the interviews that this shortage was in part related to the substantially lower wages paid to community nurses.

Discussion

Based on the interviews conducted, we conclude that SEHC successfully implemented a programme for children with complex health care needs. The principals' and nurses' comments on the programme were organized into themes related to enablers (ongoing support, monitoring, coordination of services, extensive communication, and professional development), outcomes (increased quality of life, improved access) and areas for improvement (increased awareness and funding). The enablers, or accountability processes, processes led to integrate care with health care providers becoming a part of a team focused on the child and the family.

Case managers from the CCACs were perceived by the nurses to be key members of the team. CCACs were created to deliver community based care with improved accountability and consistent quality services through the implementation of standards, best practices and management systems. In this case study, the nurses indicated that the CCACs' case managers did play a pivotal role in the provision of individualized and co-ordinated care. The case managers use a common assessment tool to determine eligibility for service and do help in the development of appropriate care plans. They focus on the student well being and help the nurses obtain the resources that they need to deliver high quality care. The nurses and principals were unambiguous about the achieved outcomes: these children with either a mental or physical disability have access to educational services because of the services that they provide. The children referred for care in school settings have multiple problems and require extensive care. Only a few years ago these children would have resided in intensive care units, with a short life expectancy. Now these children have ventilators on the back of their wheelchairs and are attending school. Access is only possible because these SEHC nurses were supported by an infrastructure and acquired complex health care skills from the Hospital for Sick Children through additional training and through other clinical experts in the field.

SEHC chose to address one of the two identified areas for improvement. Within the current funding arrangements, SEHC cannot increase salaries of nurses. However, SEHC did decide to address the lack of awareness of other professionals and the public of the SHSS programme. The school nurses received regular updates on the purpose and status of this research project and some of them were also interviewed. A poster presentation of the findings was shared at the Canadian Association of Paediatric Health Centres Conference in June 2003. A school nurse attended the conference and returned to share her learning with her colleagues at a meeting in August. She was immensely proud to have met with so many experts in paediatrics and highlighted the school programme of which she had been a part for many years. At this meeting the manager presented a video from the conference and shared the poster of the research findings. Many school nurses commented that they had not understood the programme from the broad perspective demonstrated in the poster. Additionally they had no appreciation of the quality of the whole programme but only of the small part they played as individual school nurses. This raising of esteem and sense of pride has had significant impact on the nurses' practice. This current school year 2003/04 has 0 high/low risk occurrences and 98% client satisfaction in nursing services across multiple dimensions such as cultural sensitivity, respect, mutual care planning, health teaching, nursing skills and knowledge (100% clients sampled). The nurses' enthusiasm has led to a project to publish a book of experiences in school nursing in late 2004 and each member of the school nursing team will contribute a story. The children with complex health care needs were helped through this continuous quality improvement initiative. A small acknowledgement of the care delivered by these dedicated nurses through this credible reporting helped SEHC achieve, at least partially, accountability for these children at a client level.

This success in alleviation of the fragmentation of services between sectors for children and their families was possible because several preconditions are met. These preconditions were: a shared vision, engaged stakeholders, teamwork, a focus on concrete objectives, and a monitoring of progress towards those objectives. Our findings are thus consistent with the preconditions documented in the Report of the Federal/Provincial/Territorial Advisory Committee on Population Health. The preconditions to successful intersectoral collaboration have been known for some time. Yet, examples of successful partnerships are rare. The 2001 Provincial Auditor's report on special needs education grants to school boards noted that PPM 81 was working only in a few jurisdictions . In these jurisdictions the 'respective partners treated the guidelines as policy, communicated well among themselves to ensure that their respective responsibilities were clear, and provided levels of service consistent with the needs of their school-aged populations' . The Ministry of Education responded that it was working with other ministries, agencies, community and education partners, and parents to develop service co-ordination models.

We call for a review of specialized community based paediatric services by principals, bureaucrats and health care providers. Hospital based specialized paediatric services have been recently reviewed . Community based ones have not undergone such a review. Recommendations for the delivery of all specialized paediatric health care services in Canada could be based on this case study. There was no urgent need for policy to 'catch up' with reality. Rather there is a need for the cross-sectoral development and implementation of programmes that support policies. The Canadian Public Health Association , in its submission to the Commission on the Future of Health Care in Canada entitled "A Fine Balance: A Public Health Perspective on Health System Reform," recommended the establishment of mechanisms for intersectoral collaboration. We support this recommendation but believe that to sustain these intersectoral mechanisms, additional resources are required. SEHC chose to invest in an infrastructure that benefited the nurses and the children and their families. In summary this well-designed programme properly implemented and resourced had a positive impact on children with special needs, their families and the professionals caring for them. This intersectoral protocol for children with complex health care needs in education may serve as a good model for other intersectoral integration efforts.

CHILDREN'S HEALTH HIGHLIGHTS

Children and adolescents are growing and developing, and their health care needs, use of services, and outcomes are very different from those of adults. Unlike adults, children and adolescents usually are dependent on parents and others for access to care and evaluations of the quality of that care. Furthermore, adolescents differ from younger children; they are moving from childhood to adulthood and have their own unique health care needs, preferences, and patterns of use. For these and many other reasons, a special research focus is needed to increase understanding of the issues involved in improving the delivery of health care to children and adolescents.

In 1997, six strategies for increasing the quantity and quality of child health services research (CHSR) were proposed by Christopher B. Forrest, M.D., Ph.D., of the Johns Hopkins School of Public Health, Lisa Simpson, M.B., B.Ch., Deputy Director of the Agency for Healthcare Research and Quality (AHRQ), and Carolyn Clancy, M.D., Director of AHRQ's Center for Outcomes and Effectiveness Research. In an article published in the June 11, 1997, issue of the *Journal of the American Medical Association*, they explained the need to:

1. Expand the disease orientation of health services research to include a focus on child health development.
2. Establish child-sensitive standards for setting research priorities.
3. Increase the size and capacity of the CHSR workforce.
4. Develop appropriate laboratories to study child health care.
5. Improve coordination of research funding across the Federal Government, foundations, and the private sector.
6. Enhance the research function of health care delivery in the private sector.

Finding ways to improve outcomes, quality, and access to health care for America's 70 million children and adolescents is a critical goal of health services research and a continuing priority for AHRQ. For many years, AHRQ has supported and conducted research on children's health issues. These activities are coordinated across the Agency's health services research portfolio to ensure that projects are appropriately addressed in all programme areas. This programme brief provides an overview of current AHRQ programmes, activities, and priorities in health care research for children and adolescents, as well as summaries of selected findings from recent AHRQ-supported research projects. It reflects AHRQ's commitment to build the infrastructure and capacity for child health services research and ensure that practitioners and policymakers have the knowledge and tools they need to:

— Improve child health outcomes.

— Enhance the quality of care children receive.

— Address access, use, and costs.

— Translate evidence-based research into improved clinical practice.

If copies of publications are available, that is noted under descriptions. Online information is available for AHRQ research programmes, including grant announcements and application kits. Go to Child Health to find updates on child health initiatives at AHRQ, relevant conferences and workshops, funding announcements, and more.

Acute Care/Injuries

In 2000, children and adolescents under age 18 had over 212 million ambulatory health care visits, including 49 million visits to hospital outpatient and emergency departments. Only 15 percent of visits to physicians' offices were for well-child care, while a high number of visits were for acute care. Fifty-four percent of visits to hospital emergency departments by 5-14 year olds are due to injuries, and injuries are the leading cause of death among those 1-24 years old in the United States. AHRQ's research portfolio on acute care and injuries focuses on the effectiveness, quality, and costs of care for children and adolescents.

Research in Progress

Study focuses on using evidence to enhance care for childhood illnesses

Description: Investigators are examining whether providing evidence at the point of ambulatory pediatric care will improve antibiotic use in pediatric disorders, reduce duration of therapy for acute sinusitis, reduce use of bronchodilators, and increase the use of intranasal steroids for allergic rhinitis.

Researchers are developing decision rules for use of chest x-ray to diagnose pneumonia in young children

Description: Although a relatively low proportion of chest x-rays reveal radiographic pneumonia, many young children are referred for chest-rays, resulting in unnecessary exposure to radiation and additional cost. The goal of this study is to develop decision rules that will help clinicians predict when children with lower respiratory tract infections should be sent for chest x-rays.

Analysis affirms current guidelines for treating high fever

Description: An analysis of six management strategies for a hypothetical group of 100,000 3- to 36-month-old children was conducted. Findings show that current guidelines for treating children up to age 3 who have a high fever and no obvious source of infection are the most cost effective (i.e., obtain complete blood counts and cultures, and treat children with antibiotics if the white blood cell count is equal to or greater than 15 x 109/L).

Criteria reduce unnecessary x-rays for blunt trauma victims

Description: Researchers evaluated the use of National Emergency X-Radiography Utilization Study criteria for identifying which of over 3,000 children were at low risk for cervical spine injury (CSI). Five criteria can identify pediatric blunt trauma victims who are at low risk for CSI, thereby reducing unnecessary x-rays by 20 percent.

Researchers synthesize evidence on diagnosis and treatment of sinusitis in children

Description: Researchers found little evidence on how to accurately diagnose acute sinusitis in children and note a lack of consensus on which clinical signs and symptoms are most useful for diagnosis. The various antibiotics used to treat pediatric sinusitis are equally effective; no convincing evidence supports the use of ancillary decongestants and antihistamines, and limited evidence supports the use of steroids.

Adolescent Health

Researchers have begun to target studies at the distinctive health care needs of adolescents. Establishing healthy behaviors early can reduce risks of acquiring many diseases. Recent AHRQ-funded studies have focused on such adolescent prevention topics as screening for sexually transmitted diseases and smoking cessation.

Research in Progress

Study focuses on eliminating barriers to implementation of adolescent preventive health guidelines

Description: This quality improvement (QI) intervention addresses provider and system-level barriers to delivery of preventive services to adolescents during primary care visits. The goal is to determine whether a systems intervention in a managed health care organization—including provider training and customized screening and charting tools—results in increased delivery of clinical preventive services to adolescents than the usual standard of care.

Researchers examine the role of a regular source of care for at-risk youth

Description: This study focuses on disparities in the use of physician services, the role of having a usual source of care, and the characteristics likely to result in greater use of services.

Internet learning modules for physicians may improve chlamydia screening for adolescents

Description: Study physicians will complete a year-long series of Internet learning modules that integrate case-based education with audit, feedback, and benchmarking of practice profiles. The goal is to improve chlamydia screening and treatment rates among patients aged 16-26, which should result in lower rates of pelvic inflammatory disease.

Researchers are testing an intervention for smoking cessation among rural teens

Description: The goal is to determine the usefulness of a theory-based motivational tobacco intervention for rural smokers ages 14 to 18 who seek emergency care. Researchers will develop a transportable version of the intervention for emergency facilities.

Investigators seek to improve STD screening for asymptomatic teens

Description: This QI intervention involves a small-group educational programme for clinic personnel on sexually transmitted diseases, including chlamydia. The sessions will be augmented with weekly supervision and followup to reinforce the educational content.

Recent Findings

Premature birth does not affect adolescent self-esteem

Description: Premature infants who weighed less than 2 pounds were at high risk for neurodevelopmental, cognitive, behavioral, and emotional difficulties. However, once they reached adolescence, their self-esteem was similar to that of other adolescents.

Delivery of smoking prevention/cessation services differs

Description: Researchers analyzed survey responses from pediatricians and family physicians and found that doctors used more tobacco interventions when they were familiar with the Public Health Service guidelines, spent more time with adolescent patients, and spent more time alone with patients.

Not all teens receive reproductive health services

Description: In a survey of 354 family physicians, respondents reported asking 79 percent of their adolescent patients about contraceptive use, 73 percent about condom use, 72 percent about sexual relationships, and 61 percent about sexual behavior. Female doctors and younger doctors are among those more likely to provide reproductive health screening and counseling during adolescent visits.

Providers' role in preventing alcohol problems is unclear

Description: This article summarizes what is known about adolescent alcohol use and how it can be addressed in primary care settings. Studies show that few primary care doctors follow existing guidelines that recommend yearly screening of adolescents for alcohol problems.

Adolescents accurately characterize the care they receive

Description: To develop quality measures for adolescent care, researchers recruited 400 adolescents, audiotaped their visits with physicians, and conducted phone surveys to assess their recollection of the preventive health care they received. Adolescents' recall of the care they received was good.

Researchers develop and test a taxonomy of adolescent health

Description: Researchers used four domains of health to group adolescents into 13 profile types. They also identified combinations of problems that characterize different subgroups of adolescents to develop a taxonomy of adolescent health and tested the taxonomy in four ethnically diverse groups of urban and rural youths ages 11 to 17.

Asthma

Asthma is a chronic inflammatory disease of the airways that affects approximately 5 million U.S. children a year. An estimated 400,000 of these children have moderate to severe asthma. It is the most common chronic disease of childhood, with about one-fourth of those affected being less than 5 years of age. Illness associated with asthma is on the rise, and reducing asthma-related morbidity continues to be a major objective for the U.S. Public Health Service.

Research in Progress

Study examines underuse of preventive care among black children

Description: This study is exploring the factors that contribute to the disparity between black and white children in preventive asthma care. Factors include insurance coverage, access to preventive health care, financial resources, and health beliefs.

Researchers study treatment adherence among children with cystic fibrosis and asthma

Description: The aims of this study are three-fold: (1) assess the extent of adherence problems in children with cystic fibrosis and asthma, (2) compare patterns of adherence in two pediatric pulmonary populations, and (3) identify key barriers associated with poor adherence.

Researchers explore the family effects of having a child with asthma

Description: This project will extend previous research on the impact of having a child with asthma and the burden asthma places on the family's resources, availability of care, and barriers to care.

Project underway to test the cost-effectiveness of recently developed practice guidelines for pediatric asthma

Description: This 5-year study is being conducted in three unrelated, geographically dispersed managed care settings. The researchers are evaluating educational and organizational approaches to QI for pediatric asthma care, focusing primarily on symptom assessment. They also will examine other outcomes, including functional status, health care use, and patient satisfaction.

Effects of Medicaid enrollment gaps on asthma outcomes are being studied

Description: Researchers are evaluating the effect of gaps in enrollment in Tennessee's Medicaid programme for children with asthma by studying two markers for use of asthma care—emergency room visits and hospitalizations.

Two studies explore the effects of managed care on the quality of pediatric asthma care

Description: The first study is investigating the impact of the transition from fee-for-service to managed care on quality of treatment, quality of life, and health outcomes for indigent children with asthma, as well as the impact of organizational policies on quality and outcomes. Bruce Stuart (AHRQ grant HS09950). The second study involves 2,700 children with asthma who are enrolled in nine Medicaid managed care organizations in California, Washington, and Massachusetts. Researchers are studying health plan payment mechanisms, provider profiling and incentives, and disease management programmes; patient-level features; and other variables.

Evaluation of school-based asthma care is underway

Description: Children's functional status, school days missed, and resource use are among the indicators researchers are using to evaluate the impact of using school-based health centers to deliver care for asthma.

Researchers are assessing the use of telecommunications in asthma care

Description: The researchers are assessing the effectiveness of Telephone-Linked Communications for Asthma, a computer-based system that monitors, educates, and counsels parents and children who have asthma.

Study compares two pediatric asthma management programmes

Description: Researchers are comparing a modified "easy breathing" programme with a disease management programme being used by 66 providers in 18 communities. Outcome measures will include adherence to guidelines, antiinflammatory prescription and use rates, hospitalization and ER visits, patient/family satisfaction, and quality of life.

Multisite intervention project for children with asthma may lead to improved outcomes and reduced costs

Description: Using a family-focused QI intervention for children with asthma, this study is targeting providers of care to poor, inner-city, minority youths ages 5-18 who are enrolled in a community health center-based Medicaid managed care organization. The goals are to develop a method to deliver patient-linked guideline prompts at the point of care using affordable information technology; evaluate the system's effects on the process and outcomes of pediatric asthma care; and evaluate the effects on patient outcomes of a family-focused education intervention delivered by a community health worker.

Study findings will build an asthma case-management model for Head Start

Description: The researchers are developing a pediatric asthma management model for Head Start personnel using evidence-based asthma management criteria. The goal is to improve the asthma management practices of children, parents, and staff, as well as reduce school absences and use of acute care services.

Researchers are evaluating quality improvement strategies

Description: These researchers will compare the effects of office-based QI with regular practice on processes and outcomes of care for children with asthma ages 2 to 18. Effectiveness and cost-effectiveness will be evaluated in this managed care setting.

Recent Findings

Experts develop policy recommendations for pediatric asthma

Description: Experts and leaders in childhood asthma outline policy recommendations for ensuring children are quickly diagnosed and treated, agencies are prepared to address needs, and children are safe from environmental risks that worsen asthma.

Improving medication use will reduce racial/ethnic disparities

Description: Study findings show that despite having worse asthma than white children, black and Hispanic children with similar insurance and sociodemographic characteristics are 31 and 42 percent less likely to be using inhaled antiinflammatory medication to prevent the onset or worsening of an asthma episode.

Few parents are reducing household asthma triggers

Description: In a study of 638 children with asthma, 45 percent of the parents had received written instructions about avoiding asthma triggers in their homes. Providing parents with these instructions was not associated with their efforts to do so.

Minority children get fewer medications than white children

Description: Investigators analyzed responses to questionnaires, as well as prescription, demographic, provider, and other data on 1,000 asthmatic children and their families. Black and Hispanic children received fewer bronchodilators, and Hispanic children received fewer inhaled steroids than white children (Intramural).

Mild asthma does not significantly affect quality of life

Description: Researchers analyzed asthma symptom data (based on parent and child daily logs); child-reported health status and quality-of-life (QOL) scores; and child-reported anxiety scale, depression inventory, and behavior checklist data for 339 children. Children with mild or moderate asthma do not differ in emotional functioning, symptoms, or total QOL scores, but those with moderate asthma report more activity limitations.

Tobacco smoke increases risk of respiratory diseases

Description: A literature review reveals the following: environmental tobacco smoke (ETS) increases the risk of respiratory diseases (including asthma) in children, and the home is the most important source of ETS exposure. The impact of ETS on respiratory symptoms is strongest in a child's first 2 years (Intramural).

Comorbidities led to higher use and cost of health care

Description: Records of 71,818 children enrolled in a health care group plan revealed that children with asthma were three times more likely than those without asthma to have coexisting problems. The problems (sinusitis, otitis media, and allergic rhinitis) led to higher health care use and costs.

Medicaid children use emergency departments most often

Description: Investigators studied health care use and asthma symptoms of 804 children. Medicaid children used the emergency department almost twice as often for asthma care as privately insured children.

Rates of diagnosis vary despite similarities in symptoms

Description: An asthma screening survey administered to a metropolitan and a nonmetropolitan group of American Indian and Alaska Native students found similar rates of asthma symptoms and medical visits for these symptoms. However, the students' locale, ethnicity, and socioeconomic status had a stronger effect on physician diagnosis of asthma than prevalence of asthma symptoms (Intramural).

Few children with asthma use controller medication despite guidelines

Description: Researchers conducted a 1-year study of 13,352 children with asthma who were cared for in three managed care organizations. They found that despite national guidelines recommending use of inhaled corticosteroids, few children with persistent asthma symptoms used them regularly.

Bilingual scale helps clinicians assess asthma symptoms

Description: A new Spanish-English scale for measuring the control of asthma in Latino children from low-income families has been developed and tested with parents of 234 inner-city Hispanic children with asthma (Intramural).

Factors that predict hospitalization of children with asthma have not changed over time

Description: Researchers found that teenagers and boys

were more likely than children aged 5 to 12 and girls to be hospitalized for severe respiratory distress or failure. Region of the country and hospital teaching status also were significantly associated with differences in severity of asthma among hospitalized children. The research team reviewed hospital records of more than 168,000 children in 746 hospitals in 1990 and more than 174,000 children in 811 hospitals in 1995.

Children with asthma did not improve following a pharmacist-delivered intervention

Description: Researchers assessed changes in disease control, functional status, and cost associated with a structured programme of pharmacist-delivered care for children with asthma and found no evidence that they improved in pulmonary function, functional status, quality of life, asthma management, or satisfaction with care.

Asthma affects Puerto Rican children more severely than it does other Latino children

Description: Puerto Rican children with asthma are affected by their illness significantly more than Cuban American or Mexican American children. Puerto Rican children usually have a smaller airway size, more severe inflammatory reactions, and lower birthweight than other Latino children, and their mothers are more likely to smoke cigarettes than other Hispanic mothers.

Environmental tobacco smoke contributes to early childhood asthma

Description: Data from the Third National Health and Nutrition Examination Survey (NHANES) reveal that almost half of the cases of early childhood asthma, chronic bronchitis, and wheezing result from secondhand cigarette smoke. (Intramural)

Attention Deficit/Hyperactivity Disorder

Attention deficit/hyperactivity disorder (ADHD) is a psychiatric disorder distinguished by symptoms of inattention, hyperactivity, and impulsivity, and it may be accompanied by learning disabilities, depression, anxiety, conduct disorder, and oppositional defiant disorder. ADHD is one of the most common childhood-onset disorders, with a prevalence rate of approxiately 4 percent to 12 percent for school-aged children.

AHRQ has supported the development of evidence reports on the diagnosis and treatment of ADHD, research on the costs associated with the disorder, and efforts to improve quality of care for ADHD.

Research in Progress

Workshops will facilitate applications of research to practice

Description: This conference grant supports a series of learning opportunities to improve care for children with ADHD. The goal is to promote the translation of the evidence about the diagnosis and treatment of ADHD into clinical practice.

Study examines use of computers in caring for children with ADHD.

Description: The researchers will develop and evaluate a computerized system for laptop use in the examining room to improve the care of children with ADHD.

New tools are being developed to help families cope with ADHD

Description: Researchers are developing tools for families with children who have ADHD to help them coordinate the child's care and inform parents, teachers, and health providers.

Recent Findings

Costs are similar for ADHD and asthma

Description: Data from the 1996 Medical Expenditure Panel Survey reveal annual health care costs for children with ADHD and asthma were $479 and $437 more than the those of the general population of children.

Evidence report focuses on children with ADHD.

Description: Researchers assessed the effectiveness and long- and short-term safety of pharmacological and nonpharmacological interventions for ADHD.

AHRQ technical review focuses on the screening tests used to diagnose ADHD

Description: The researchers identified several rating scales that effectively discriminate between ADHD children and normal controls. Broad-band behavior rating scales were ineffective in identifying ADHD children, as were imaging procedures (CT, CAT scan, MRI) and neurological screening tests.

HEALTH INFORMATION TECHNOLOGY IN CHILDREN'S HEALTH CARE

AHRQ's Focus on Child and Adolescent Health

The Agency for Healthcare Research and Quality provides support for a broad portfolio of research projects focused on health care—including the use of health IT—for America's 70 million children and adolescents. Findings from AHRQ-supported research on children's health help to guide clinical decisionmaking, provide essential information for health care policymakers, and fill the gaps that exist in evidence-based information on the health care needs of children and adolescents. The rapidly growing and changing field of health IT is no exception. Health IT is emerging as a key element to better, safer, and more effective health care for all patients. AHRQ has a long-standing commitment to support research on the development, testing, use, and impediments to implementation of health IT, as well as the effects of health IT on quality and safety.

This programme brief summarizes the Agency's efforts in support of using health IT in children's health care, including findings from AHRQ-funded research, conferences, and ongoing and recently completed research projects. Select for *more information* about AHRQ's research on child and adolescent, health and health information technology, and other topics.

AHRQ-Supported Activities

Health information technology (health IT) holds great promise for improving the quality, safety, efficiency, and effectiveness of health care for all patients, including children and adolescents. In addition to improving care for patients and giving providers and health systems a powerful tool for reducing errors, health IT has the potential to produce savings of up to 10 percent of the country's total annual spending on health care.

Researchers and policymakers are just beginning to explore and understand the very important role that health IT will play in the Nation's health care system in the coming years. For example, we already know that health IT has the potential to improve patient safety, enhance communication between providers and patients, and reduce inappropriate care.

We need to know much more about using health IT to its fullest potential to improve health care in America. In order to do this, we also have to understand the barriers and challenges that are impediments to implementation of health IT so that we can identify ways to overcome them.

Research Findings

Five technologies are expected to improve patient safety for children

For an AHRQ-supported conference on pediatric patient safety research, investigators reviewed the use of information technology in children's health care and concluded that five technologies have the greatest potential to improve patient safety:

1. Care provider order entry with decision support.
2. Guideline-based documentation tools.
3. Internet-based disease management resources.
4. Teleconsultation.
5. Electronic health records other than order entry or documentation tools.

Use of a Computer-based Documentation (CBD) Tool Does not Change Parent and Physician Communication

Researchers investigated the impact of a CBD tool on parent and physician satisfaction with a pediatric health maintenance encounter. There was no change in overall parent or physician satisfaction in the areas of communication and physician helpfulness. There was no correlation between physician and parent satisfaction or between physician satisfaction and pattern of CBD use. However, there was a strong correlation between physicians' satisfaction and the extent to which they found CBD helpful.

Telemedicine Reduces Absence from Child Care Due to Illness

A telemedicine model for diagnosis and treatment of common acute problems used both real-time and store-and-forward information exchange between a child and telemedicine assistant in child care and an office-based telemedicine clinician. Absences due to acute illness during weeks with telemedicine were less than half those that occurred during weeks without telemedicine. Researchers concluded that telemedicine holds substantial potential to reduce the impact of illness on the health and education of children, time lost from work by parents, and absenteeism in the economy.

Telephone-Linked Communication (TLC) System Supports Care of Children with Persistent Asthma

These researchers developed and tested an information system designed to integrate patient health information across multiple domains to support the monitoring and care of children with persistent asthma. Used in a multi-specialty group practice, this system includes three primary components:

6. A patient-centered, telephone-linked communication system.
7. A Web-based alert reporting and nurse case-management system.
8. Electronic medical record-based provider communication to support clinical decisionmaking at the point of care.

According to the authors, this system offers a new level of connectivity for health information, IT-enabled nurse case managers, and the delivery of longitudinal data to clinicians to support the care of children with persistent asthma.

Prioritizing Computer-Based Prompts for Preventive Services

These authors describe two approaches to prioritizing prompts for child preventive services: one approach involves a static, global prioritization across all preventive services; the second approach uses influence diagrams to prioritize prompts based on individual patient data. The latter approach is still under development. Both methods are labor-intensive and require a combination of epidemiologic data and expert judgment.

Researchers Examine User Acceptance of a Clinical Computer System in Two Pediatric Practices

Data for this qualitative study were gathered through interviews with staff, clinical observations, and review of system implementation records. Five months after implementation, Practice A continued to use the system, but Practice B had abandoned it because it was unacceptable to the users. Five main themes were identified relative to differences in user acceptance:

9. Benefits versus expense of system use varied.
10. Organizational cultures differed.
11. Staff relationship with practices differed.
12. Post-implementation experiences differed.
13. Transfer of technology from the academic center to private practice proved challenging in Practice B.

The findings indicate a need for the development and validation of tools to measure health care organizational climate and readiness for change.

Researchers Investigate Challenges of Automating a Real-Time Clinical Practice Guideline

The goal of this study was to describe the types of problems encountered during implementation of a Web-based clinical practice guideline to manage hyperbilirubinemia in newborn infants. The researchers conducted a formative assessment of an automated guideline in a large-scale implementation in primary-care clinics and offices, inpatient clinics, and an emergency department affiliated with an academic children's hospital. They found that many existing guidelines are not amenable to straightforward implementation in automated systems. However, strategies to increase the efficacy of the automated guidelines included guideline modifications, as well as careful consideration of the flow of clinical work.

Mining Association Rules from a Pediatric Primary Care Decision Support System

For this study, researchers applied an unsupervised data mining algorithm to a database containing data on over 30,000 visits collected at the point of care for clinical decision support. The data set was taken from the Child Health Improvement Programme, a preventive services tracking system at the University of North Carolina. Researchers used a previously described pattern discovery algorithm to extract 2nd and 3rd order association rules from the data and reviewed the literature to see if the associations had been described before. The algorithm discovered 16 2nd order associations and 103 3rd order associations. The 3rd order associations contained no new information, while the 2nd order associations demonstrated a covariance among a range of health risk behaviors. Additionally, use of the algorithm revealed that both exposure to tobacco smoke and chronic cardiopulmonary disease are associated with failure on developmental screens. These relationships were attributed to underlying poverty. This research demonstrated the ability of unsupervised data mining by rule association on sparse clinical data to discover clinically important associations. However, many associations may be previously known or explained by confounding variables.

Health IT Can Empower Parents and Children to Make Informed Health Care Decisions

These authors present examples of interactive

information technologies that facilitate information sharing and empower children and families: the electronic pediatric personal medical record (PPMR), customized health information systems, and interactive physician offices with E-mail and telemedicine capabilities. The exact form of an electronic PPMR is still evolving, but ultimately it may resemble currently available personal financial management programmes. It could reside on an individual's personal computer, commercial Web site, or other commercial system, and part of the record may exist as smart cards or electronic dogtags. One-half of Internet users say that they would like to E-mail their doctors. E-mail allows continuous access to the health care system for non-urgent matters such as care coordination, augmented screening, symptom monitoring, and disease self-management. Telemedicine also holds great promise for patient care. For example, video conferencing could benefit home care personnel and family caregivers of children with medically complex needs for whom transportation to multiple specialists is costly and burdensome.

AHRQ-Funded Research Projects

Improving the Safety of Blood Product Transfusions in Children

This project involves a probabilistic risk assessment (PRA) of blood product transfusion practices in children so that opportunities to reduce errors and improve safety for other low-frequency, high-impact processes can be identified. The PRA tool is a hybrid between process analysis and decision support methods used in high-risk industries. Using hospital discharge data from AHRQ's Healthcare Cost and Utilization Project and the Pediatric Health Information System databases, the researchers will determine the proportion of hospitalizations in which blood product transfusions are administered and describe patient characteristics associated with transfusions.

Valuation of Primary Care-Integrated Telehealth

Health-e-Access is a commercially available technology that enables clinicians to evaluate and treat ill children at distant child care or school sites. Factors affecting its widespread use include physician acceptance, practice implementation, and insurance reimbursement. These key issues are being investigated in two demonstration projects (Study A and Study B) in 9 schools and 13 child care programmes in the Rochester, NY, area. Study A is focusing on the impact of telehealth on use and costs at the facility and child levels. Study B is assessing integration in primary care by measuring impact on continuity of care and adherence to well-child visit schedules and immunization rates.

Kenneth McConnochie, Principal Investigator, University of Rochester, Rochester, NY. AHRQ grant HS15165, project period 9/30/04-9/29/07.

ParentLink: Better and Safer Emergency Care for Children

In this study, researchers are:

1. Evaluating the completeness and accuracy of information on symptoms, disease/condition, medications, and allergies generated by parents using ParentLink versus information documented by emergency department (ED) physicians and nurses.
2. Measuring the impact of ParentLink on ED patient safety and quality, specifically the error rate for ordering and prescribing medications during ED care and the percent of ED visits that adhere to national evidence-based guidelines.

Improving Pediatric Safety and Quality with Health Care IT

In this study, researchers are assessing changes in patient experience of care using a modified CAHPS® survey to evaluate the influence of:

3. Weight-based dosing on pediatric adverse drug events.
4. A test result tracking system on appropriate followup of ordered tests.
5. Automated reminders on symptom monitoring and medications for children with asthma and attention deficit disorder.

This study includes inner-city minority communities, especially Hispanic and African-American populations.

Showing Health Information Value in a Community Network

The goal of this 3-year project is to assess the costs and benefits of health IT in an established community-wide network of academic, private, and public health care facilities. The network was created to share clinical information for the purpose of population-based care management of over 16,000 Medicaid beneficiaries in Durham County, NC. Researchers are evaluating the impact of information-driven interventions on care quality, patient safety, and costs. The majority of patients in this study are minority children (African-American, Hispanic, and other ethnicities) and women.

Improving Safety and Quality with Integrated Technology

The aims of this project are to:

6. Demonstrate the value of an integrated outpatient and inpatient health IT system to improve quality of care and safety for women and infants, using group B streptococcus (GBS) prevention as the test case.
7. Demonstrate the value of an outpatient alert system to increase GBS screening.
8. Perform a cost-benefit analysis to assess the economic

impact of implementing the integrated health IT system.

Impact of Health Information Technology on Clinical Care

This study has two principal aims. The first is to determine the impact on quality and safety of ambulatory health IT for patients with one or more of five chronic diseases (asthma, coronary artery disease, congestive heart failure, diabetes mellitus, and hypertension). This is being done by evaluating measures of drug use, laboratory monitoring, and physiologic disease control. The second goal is to determine the impact of ambulatory health IT on resource use for the same patients by estimating the rates of office visits, ED visits, and hospitalizations. A large number of children with asthma and fewer children with diabetes are included in this study, as well as women and minorities.

Improving Quality of Care for Children with Special Needs

The goal of this study was development of a database to include diagnosis, health records, and educational information on children with special health care needs in the Tennessee Child Health Profile. The project included low-income, minority children.

Can Hand-Held Technology Reduce Errors in ADHD Care?

This randomized controlled trial was conducted in three primary care practices. The researchers developed and evaluated a computerized system for laptop use in the examining room as an extension of an existing in-house prescribing system. The goal was to improve the care of children with attention-deficit/hyperactivity disorder.

Creating Online NICU Networks to Educate, Consult and Team

The goal of this study was to develop, implement, and evaluate a cooperative effort using health IT to facilitate a continuum of appropriate medical and developmental care for infants most at risk for long-term neurodevelopmental problems. High-risk infants, including Asians and African Americans from birth to 24 months, were represented in this study.

El Dorado County Safety Network Technology Project

The goal of this study was to integrate the Network's "Access Product" to improve care for indigent and low-income children and families. Three approaches were used: one, outreach and study enrollment for children eligible for public insurance; two, access to quality health care services for children not eligible for public insurance up to 300 percent of the poverty level; and three, access to health care for families employed by local small businesses unable to provide coverage for their workers. The safety net population included in this study was rural indigent, low-income, uninsured, and underinsured minorities, women, and children.

Electronic Records to Improve Care for Children

The aims of this project are to:

9. Implement a shared, electronic health record for health care providers in pediatric primary care, school health, specialty care, and emergency medicine.
10. Demonstrate improvements in quality of care for children with asthma.
11. Clarify organizational barriers and factors that enhance IT acceptance.
12. Provide administrative and technical elements of a community-wide health network infrastructure that can be further extended to additional health partners, including academic health center clinics, community

health centers, hospital emergency departments, and inpatient facilities.

This study involves an inner-city, multiethnic group of children and women and includes minority physicians and nurse practitioners who practice at partner sites.

Comprehensive IT Solutions for Quality and Patient Safety

This pediatric health care system is implementing a series of health information technologies to improve patient safety and quality, as well as increase efficiency of all operaticns. Four related technologies focusing on pharmacy are involved: an inpatient pharmacy system, an electronic medication administration record, a bar coding system, and a computerized provider order entry system. Study participants include women, minorities, and inner-city children using Medicaid.

Creating an Evidence Base for Vision Rehabilitation

The goals of this study are to:

13. Train staff in using best-practice protocols.
14. Install electronic vision rehabilitation records at three nonprofit vision rehabilitation agencies.
15. Determine, build, and pilot the electronic interface between government agencies, private rehabilitation agencies, and primary care providers.
16. Validate the system's logic and predictive ability.
17. Construct and populate a national benchmarking database with outcome-measurement data from pilot sites.

This will result in the first vision rehabilitation evidence base for best treatment practice. This study includes patients aged 6 months and older.

Colorado Connecting Communities—Health Information Collaborative (C3-HIC)

The purpose of this project is to implement State-wide information and communications technologies that will allow clinicians at the point of care to access patient information from other clinical data repositories.

Conferences, Expert Meetings, and Editorials

National Child Health Data Standards Workgroup Meeting

AHRQ, the Florida Initiative for Children's Healthcare Quality (FLICHQ), and the National Initiative for Children's Health Quality (NICHQ) sponsored an expert meeting on April 5, 2005, to kick off the Child Health Information Technology Standards Project. The goal of this 2-year initiative is to further the development, testing, and advancement of data standards specific to children's health care. The project components are:

1. The establishment of a National Child Data Standards Workgroup.
2. The commissioning of four papers that discuss the issues of using health IT for children's health.
3. Hosting a national expert meeting.
4. Establishing a technical expert panel charged with developing a draft set of data standards for one child health topic within 18 months.

The All Children's Hospital Foundation of Pinellas County, FL, provided a grant in support of this project.

Information Technology for Children's Health and Health Care: Beginning to Ask the Needed Questions

AHRQ and the American Academy of Pediatrics' Center for Child Health Research sponsored a meeting held September 21-22, 2000, of experts and stakeholders to identify the special information needs of pediatric care and health services research questions related to the use of health IT in children's health care. Several articles summarized here facilitated discussions at the meeting and were subsequently published. They are:

Research and implementation agenda recommendations. The group proposed a research agenda to address both effectiveness and costs of information technology, with special consideration for the needs of children; the development and evaluation of clinical decision support in pediatric settings; supplementation of vocabulary standards with pediatrics-specific terminology; and improvement in health care access for children using telemedicine. Recommendations included rapid implementation of features in electronic health information systems that support pediatric patient care.

Barriers that impede the adoption of pediatric information technology: These authors reviewed the literature to summarize barriers that are likely to affect the adoption of health IT by pediatric professionals. They conclude that some barriers may represent a challenge and others—such as the lack of knowledge about the uses of health IT—are more easily resolved. Efforts to overcome these barriers should begin in earnest and should include educating stakeholders in the care of children and adolescents, as well as improving the knowledge about various technologies available to support pediatric and adolescent health care.

Information Technology and the Future of Child Health Care—A Revolution is Occurring: In this editorial, the author discusses the revolution in communications and information technology both inside and outside homes and workplaces. This revolution will have broad influence on the practice of pediatrics, and it holds great promise to improve the quality of health care, reduce medical errors, enhance the knowledge of parents and their effective involvement in their children's health care, and improve child and adolescent health.

4

Health Care Disparities & Public Health Services

NATIONAL HEALTHCARE DISPARITIES REPORT

The National Healthcare Disparities Report, developed by the Agency for Healthcare Research and Quality (AHRQ), is the first national comprehensive effort to measure differences in access and use of health care services by various populations. The report includes a broad set of performance measures that can serve as baseline views of differences in the use of services. The report presents data on differences in the use of services, access to health care, and impressions of quality for seven clinical conditions, including cancer, diabetes, end-stage renal disease, heart disease, HIV and AIDS, mental health, and respiratory disease as well as data on maternal and child health, nursing home and home health care, and patient safety. It also examines differences in use of services by priority populations.

This historic report, the first annual report on healthcare disparities, is intended to provide a balanced summary of the state of disparities in the United States. It will demonstrate that disparities exist for many Americans and improvement is possible. Rather than offer a series of snapshots of disparities from individual research studies, this report provides a comprehensive view of the scope and characteristics of differences in health care quality and access associated with patient race, ethnicity, income, education, and place of residence. To date, no report has provided extensive cross-group comparisons that could provide a national roadmap to focused efforts to reduce disparities. Demographic trends indicate that the number of Americans who are vulnerable to suffering the effects of heath care disparities will rise over the next half century. Current data show that some ethnic minorities, as well as low-income families of whatever race or ethnicity, tend to be in poorer health than other Americans. "The evidence of the damaging health consequences of racial and ethnic disparities in health care continues to be overwhelming," says John W. Rowe, M.D., Chairman, President and CEO of Aetna. Gaps in income between the richest and poorest households in America are also widening. Additionally, some racial and ethnic minorities are growing at a much more rapid pace than the majority white population. Nearly 1 in 2 Americans will be a member of a racial or ethnic minority—i.e., black, Hispanic, Asian, or American Indian—by the year 2050. Clearly, these trends pose a daunting challenge for policymakers and the health care system.

Health Care Disparities

The word "disparity" can be defined as "the condition or fact of being unequal, as in age, rank, or degree." Synonyms for disparity include *inequality*, *unlikeness*, *disproportion*, and *difference*. While disparity in health care has been closely associated with equity, there are several potential reasons for the differences observed at the individual level. For example, a patient may receive fewer medications because of differences in underlying disease processes, individual choice, systemic barriers to obtaining needed medications, or some combination of these reasons. When we observe differences in health care for different populations, it may not be possible to clarify causal pathways directly. The purpose of this report is to describe differences in quality of and access to health care to help identify disparities in health outcomes that may be responsive to improvements in health care. Disparities are most easily identified when there is a clear reference point for what is appropriate and reasonable to expect. While there may be uncertainty regarding many aspects of clinical care, the quality measures presented here have been developed around health care interventions for which there is sound scientific evidence of effectiveness and for which there is a professional consensus and expectation that these services would be provided to all patients. Even after consideration of variation in patients' medical conditions and severity of illness, there should be little deviation from specific quality measures associated with population.

Access to health care is a prerequisite to obtaining quality care. However, dimensions of access vary in predicting an individual's likelihood of receiving care that has been shown to improve health outcomes. For use of services, patient-reported experience of care, and structural issues such as transportation, there is limited scientific consensus regarding which measures are most responsive to system improvements. In addition, the most important factors may not be consistent across communities and populations. This report presents a broad array of differences related to access, use, and patient experience of care by racial, ethnic, socioeconomic, and geographic groups, based on valid measures. Many of the differences presented here are large and worrisome; indeed, some will argue, quite reasonably, that they constitute evidence of disparity, irrespective of a clear relationship to health outcomes. Further evaluation of these data should prove helpful in assessing current efforts to address important disparities in access to care. At this juncture, it may be useful to comment briefly on the complexity of the task. First, as noted above, many factors may lead to differences in health care, especially with respect to aggregate measures of use. These include different underlying rates of illness due to genetic predisposition, local environmental conditions, or lifestyle choices. There are differences in the care-seeking behaviour of patients, which vary due to differing cultural beliefs, linguistic barriers, degree of trust of health care providers, or variations in the predisposition to seek timely care. In addition, the availability of care is dependent upon such factors as the ability to pay for care (directly or through insurance coverage), the location, management and delivery of health care services, clinical uncertainty, and health care practitioner beliefs, among others. Second, there may be differing perspectives regarding the appropriate division of responsibility between the individual, the public sector, and the private sector. Third, to the extent that defining a difference establishes it as a priority for action, it is not clear that reliance upon a consistent numerical threshold is appropriate. For some measures reported here, a small differential could be critical; for others, a differential may not be critical unless it is very large. It will be important to take into account the impact on patients of the differential. Last, how the patient characteristics assessed in this report—race, ethnicity, income, education, place of residence, age, and others—affect quality of and access to health care are both independent and additive. This first National Healthcare Disparities Report presents descriptive information for each but does not assess which characteristics are most important for improving health care.

National Healthcare Disparities Report

Public Law 106-129, the Healthcare Research and Quality Act of 1999, directed the Agency for Healthcare Research and Quality (AHRQ) to develop two annual reports: a National Healthcare Quality Report (NHQR) and this National Healthcare Disparity Report (NHDR). The directive for this report, now contained in section 903(a)(6) of the Public Health Service Act, requires that this annual report tracks "prevailing disparities in health care delivery as they relate to racial factors and socioeconomic factors in priority populations." With guidance from the Institute of Medicine, AHRQ developed a common conceptual framework for both reports and, in fact, a focus on quality is at the heart of both reports. As the IOM noted in its report, *Guidance for the National Healthcare Disparities Report*, the "plan to make health care quality a major focus of this report...is appropriate since disparities often represent an 'inequality in quality.'" The conceptual framework for the NHQR focuses on safety, effectiveness, patient centeredness, and timeliness, with equity as a cross-cutting dimension. Equity, as envisioned by the IOM, is "the provision of health care of equal quality based solely on need and clinical factors." The NHDR provides a full and comprehensive expansion of the equity dimension. Therefore, these highly linked reports are being released simultaneously and readers are urged to review both reports together to develop a more comprehensive snapshot of the performance of our health care system, its strengths, and areas that should serve as a focal point for future improvement. The performance measures underlying the two reports will be used to monitor the Nation's progress toward improved health care delivery.

This first NHDR provides a national overview of racial, ethnic, and socioeconomic disparities in health care in the general U.S. population and among "priority populations" to contribute to the public dialogue on how to improve health care delivery for all Americans. These "priority populations, are defined in AHRQ's authorizing statute (section 901 (c) of the Public Health Service Act) as encompassing both specific population groups as well as geographically-defined groups. In accordance with these guidelines, the NHDR includes data and analysis on the following: low-income groups; racial and ethnic minority groups; women; children; the elderly; individuals with special health care needs, the disabled, people in need of long-term care, people requiring end-of-life care, and place of residence (e.g., rural communities). Although other demographic groups may also suffer from health care disparities, they are beyond the scope of this report. It is important to note that this report is unique in providing a systematic overview of differences in health care for both racial and ethnic groups as well as by socioeconomic status.

This is the first comprehensive look at differences by socioeconomic groups. Although not designed to measure the progress of any one programme or policy, the data and analyses presented in the report are intended to provide a convenient and comprehensive source of information spanning a broad range of health care disparity issues. "We need an annual report to measure whether we are making progress in ending racial disparities in health care and improving the quality of life for all Americans," said U.S. Representative Danny K. Davis (D-IL) when introducing the amendment calling for the NHDR. He added: "This amendment is designed to try and make sure that we have adequate and accurate information on which to base policy and budgetary decisions."

Objectives of the First Report

A vital step in the effort to eliminate health care disparities is the systematic collection and analysis of health care data. This will help policymakers and researchers discern the areas of greatest need, monitor trends over time, and identify successful programmes for addressing those needs. This first NHDR builds on and seeks to complement existing work in the area of disparities, notably *Healthy People 2010* and IOM's 2002 report, *Unequal Treatment: Confronting Racial and Ethnic Disparities in Healthcare*. Yet those efforts differ from the NHDR in substantive ways. The elimination of disparities in health is a goal of *Healthy People 2010*. Since the extent to which disparities in health care contribute to overall disparities in health remains unknown, the NHDR complements HP 2010 by focusing on prevailing disparities in health care delivery. Disparities in health care can only be interpreted within the context of disparities in health. Eliminating disparities in health care is a logical method for eliminating associated disparities in health.

Unequal Treatment extensively documents health care disparities in the United States by race and ethnicity. The IOM's examination finds that disparities in health care are substantial, even after accounting for characteristics typically associated with disparities, such as health insurance coverage and income. But while *Unequal Treatment* demonstrates definitively that racial and ethnic disparities in health care exist, it does not measure the magnitude of the problem from a national perspective. The report also does not address disparities in access to health care or disparities related to socioeconomic position. In contrast, the NHDR examines national disparities in both the ability of Americans to access health care and in the quality of health care. It includes an analysis of disparities related to socioeconomic position as well as to race and ethnicity, and attempts to capture the relationship between race/ethnicity and socioeconomic position. The report provides baseline data from which we may be able to measure the effect of national initiatives to reduce disparities.

Key Findings

The NHDR provides seven key findings to policymakers, clinicians, health system administrators, and community leaders who seek to use this information to improve health care services for all populations:

1. Inequality in quality persists.
2. Disparities come at a personal and societal price.
3. Differential access may lead to disparities in quality.
4. Opportunities to provide preventive care are frequently missed.
5. Knowledge of why disparities exist is limited.
6. Improvement is possible.
7. Data limitations hinder targeted improvement efforts.

Inequality in Quality Exists

This report presents the most comprehensive national picture confirms that there is significant inequality in quality in the United States. While selected research studies have documented disparities in healthcare services, these examinations were often limited to specific populations with specific conditions. By using nationally available data sets, a national view on healthcare disparities is provided. This first report clearly demonstrates that racial, ethnic, and socioeconomic disparities are national problems that affect health care at all points in the process, at all sites of care, and for all medical conditions—in fact, disparities are pervasive in our health care system. Our conclusions bring us closer to understanding why, where, and how disparities occur—essential knowledge for devising and targeting programmes to eliminate these inequities. While disparities in health care potentially affect all Americans and individuals from of any group, they are not uniformly distributed across populations. We are only beginning to understand the magnitude of differential burden of illness in populations with special health care needs, such as minority children and poor patients with disabling chronic illnesses. Geography can play an important mitigating role in healthcare disparities. Remote rural populations, for example, are clearly at risk for having worse access and receiving poorer quality care.

Examples from the NHDR:

— Minorities are more likely to be diagnosed with late-stage breast cancer and colorectal cancer compared with whites.

— Patients of lower socioeconomic position are less likely to receive recommended diabetic services and more likely to be hospitalized for diabetes and its complications.

— When hospitalized for acute myocardial infarction, Hispanics are less likely to receive optimal care.

— Many racial and ethnic minorities and persons of lower socioeconomic position are more likely to die from HIV. Minorities also account for a disproportionate share of new AIDS cases.

— The use of physical restraints in nursing homes is higher among Hispanics and Asian/Pacific Islanders compared with non-Hispanic whites.

— Blacks and poorer patients have higher rates of avoidable hospital admissions (i.e., hospitalisations for health conditions that, in the presence of comprehensive primary care, rarely require hospitalisation).

Disparities Come at a Personal and Societal Price

Health care disparities are costly. Poorly managed care or missed diagnoses result in expensive and avoidable complications. As discussed in Unequal Treatment: "to the extent that minority beneficiaries of publicly funded health programmes are less likely to receive high quality care, these beneficiaries—as well as the taxpayers that support public health care programmes—may face higher future health care costs." The personal cost of disparities can lead to significant morbidity, disability, and lost productivity at the individual level. At the societal level, distal costs follow from proximal opportunities that were missed to intervene and reduce burden of illness. For example, end-stage renal disease may result from longstanding poorly controlled diabetes. The highly morbid and highly costly condition could potentially be avoided with access to indicated services and effective management of diabetes.

Examples from the NHDR:

— Without screening, cancers may not be detected until they grow large or metastasize to distant sites and cause symptoms. Such late stage cancers are usually associated with more limited treatment options and poorer survival. Minorities and persons of lower socioeconomic status are less likely to receive cancer screening services and more likely to have late stage cancer when the disease is diagnosed.

— Persons with diabetes of lower socioeconomic position are less likely to receive recommended diabetic services and more likely to be hospitalized for diabetes and its complications.

— Many racial and ethnic minorities and persons of lower socioeconomic position are less likely to receive recommended immunisations for influenza and pneumococcal pneumonia, the most common type of pneumonia. Once hospitalized, some ethnic and racial minorities, as well as lower income patients, suffer worse quality of care for pneumonia. These differential rates of vaccination and hospitalisation present opportunities for provider-based and community-based interventions to reduce disparities.

Differential Access May Lead to Disparities in Quality

Access to healthcare is an important prerequisite to obtaining quality care. Some access barriers, whether perceived or actual, can result in adverse health outcomes. Patients may perceive barriers to delay seeking needed care, resulting in presentation of illness at a later, less treatable stage of illness. For example, a usual source of care can serve as a navigator to the healthcare system and an advocate to obtain needed evidence-based preventive and health care services. Of the major measures of access, the lack of health insurance has significant consequences. Avoidable hospitalisations are a good example of the link between access and disparities in quality of care. These hospitalisations may reflect, in part, the adequacy of primary care. When health care needs are not met by the primary health care system, rates of avoidable admissions may rise. In contrast, perceived problems with specialty referral do not have clear clinical consequences.

Examples from the NHDR:

- — Many racial and ethnic minorities and individuals of lower socioeconomic status are less likely to have a usual source of care.
- — Hispanics and people of lower socioeconomic status are more likely to report unmet health care needs
- — While most of the population has health insurance, racial and ethnic minorities are less likely to report health insurance compared with whites. Lower income persons are also less likely to report insurance compared with higher income persons.

— Higher rates of avoidable admissions by blacks and lower socioeconomic position persons may be explained, in part, by lower receipt of routine care by these populations.

Opportunities to Provide Preventive Care are Frequently Missed

Our healthcare system continues to emphasize care that occurs after an illness occurs, rather than preventive services that could potentially prevent the illness or reduce the burden of disease. While the NHQR documents that this is a pervasive issue for all Americans, there are significant disparities in the use of evidence-based preventive services for certain populations. For example, while smoking remains the single most preventable cause of mortality, rates of smoking cessation counseling during hospitalisation are only 40 percent. For blacks, this rate of smoking cessation counseling is only 29%. Given the significant impact on morbidity, mortality, outcomes, and costs of care, efforts to target preventive services to populations most at risk would be a critical aspect of an improvement strategy to decrease disparities. Examples of missed opportunities for preventive services from the NHDR:

— Blacks and persons of lower socioeconomic status tend to have higher rates of death from cancer. While rates of cancer death may reflect a variety of factors not associated with health care such as genetic disposition, diet, and lifestyle, screening and early treatment of cancers can lead to reductions in mortality.

— Many racial and ethnic minorities and persons of lower socioeconomic position are less likely to receive screening and treatment for cardiac risk factors. The combination of lower screening and effective treatment of risk factors, such as smoking among the uninsured, lend themselves to quality improvement initiatives that can potentially reduce heart disease disparities among populations at risk.

— Many racial and ethnic minorities and persons of lower socioeconomic position are less likely to receive childhood immunisations.

— Many racial and ethnic minorities and individuals of lower socioeconomic status are less likely to receive recommended immunisations for influenza and pneumococcal disease.

Knowledge of Why Disparities Exist is Limited

There are complicated interrelationships between race, ethnicity, and socioeconomic status that may result in healthcare disparities. While we may have sufficient data about racial disparities by race and ethnicity, it is difficult to tease out the individual contributions of race, income or education to these differences. For example, we found significantly lower rates of smoking cessation offered to minority patients. However, we cannot determine how much these differences are affected by different levels of patient income, education, or types of insurance. While the relationships between these factors may seem theoretical, a better understanding of the underlying factors that result in disparities could better target improvement efforts aimed at reducing disparities. Further research may help to sort out these issues for future reports. The report cannot tell us what factors are causally related to healthcare disparities, though it does identify factors that may be related to disparities. Examples from the NHDR include:

— Many racial and ethnic groups, as well as poor and less educated patients, are more likely to have report poor communication with their physicians.

- Many racial and ethnic minorities and poor patients report more problems with some aspects of the patient-provider relationships.
- Many racial and ethnic minorities and lower income patients report more difficult patient-provider relationships.
- Asians, Hispanics, and those of lower socioeconomic status have greater difficulty accessing health care information, including information on prescription drugs.

Improvement is Possible

While the report offers a sobering view of healthcare disparities, there are some positive findings that suggest that targeted improvement efforts could significantly reduce healthcare disparities. There are some notable exceptions that demonstrate *what is possible*.

- While blacks and poor patients are more likely to present with later stage cancers with higher death rates, black women have higher screening rates for cervical cancer and no evidence of later stage cervical cancer presentation. While it would not be possible to demonstrate a causal link, the significant investment in community-based cancer screening and outreach programmes for cervical cancer may be responsible for the lack of disparity.
- Quality improvement efforts have resulted in demonstrable reductions in black-white differences in hemodialysis. A targeted intervention within a quality improvement culture may offer important lessons in disparity reduction.
- Black patients are more likely to receive blood pressure monitoring without any disparity in blood

pressure management. A greater perceived risk for significant cardiovascular disease among blacks may result in appropriately increased screening rates and treatment for risk factors. Directed public education campaigns about cardiac risk factors and the importance of an activated patient may play an important role in the lower observed rate of cardiac disparities among blacks.

When detailed data are available at the most actionable level, such as population subgroups, the efficiency of quality improvement efforts can be enhanced. For example, the subpopulation data from the California Health Interview Survey (CHIS) would allow more targeted prevention efforts directed at Asians over age 50 in need of colorectal cancer screening. The information on language spoken at home provides a far more precise target population—Asians who do not speak English were 20% less likely to undergo colorectal cancer screening than their English-speaking Asian counterparts. The disparities report can also serve to identify the best "performers," learn from their experiences and disseminate the lessons learned to other communities. Community-based participatory research has numerous examples of communities working to improve quality overall, while reducing healthcare disparities for vulnerable populations.

Data Limitations Hinder Targeted Improvement Efforts

This report provides the most comprehensive and in-depth information on health care quality and access for priority populations available. However, because the focus of the report is national and populations of interest vary across communities, it may not be possible to extrapolate national findings to any one community. Our first report on the current state of health care disparities in the nation has relied heavily on federal data collection sources. Although many health care organisations do not routinely collect data on patient characteristics, several private initiatives are currently underway, and it is clear that successful improvement efforts often occur at State and local levels. The National Healthcare Disparities Report should help to provide the impetus and tools for public and private entities that are interested in measuring and monitoring progress to eliminate disparities. While beyond the scope of this first annual report, future reports should also help to communicate successful interventions that may reduce the burden of healthcare disparities in our nation. The report also raises important questions regarding public reporting of data by race, ethnicity, and socioeconomic status. For example, expanding current public reporting initiatives to display results stratified by patient characteristics (e.g., race, ethnicity, income, education, place of residence) has been suggested. However, given sample size constraints, public reporting is not feasible at the level of individual providers. Some studies also suggest that many patients are reluctant to report income. Should national data collection efforts include stratification by race, ethnicity, income and education? Should aggregation for public reporting be required at certain levels, such as local or regional? Finally, though existing national data are useful to address many disparities, there are significant gaps. While improved data would help measure disparities, the field would also benefit from more robust measures that would improve our understanding of the underlying mechanisms and causal paths that result in disparities.

PUBLIC HEALTH SERVICE HOSPITAL DISTRICT: RESIDENTIAL AND EDUCATIONAL COMMUNITY

Planning Concept

The historic complex of buildings at the former Public Health Service Hospital will be rehabilitated to accommodate new uses, with a preference for residential and educational uses. Important natural resources, including habitat for rare and unique plant and wildlife species, will be protected and enhanced. Non-historic structures may be removed, and replacement construction could be considered in the future. New construction would be carefully sited and designed to enhance the serene, campus-like historic setting.

Residential and Educational Uses are Preferred for the Public Health Service Hospital District

Character, Land Use, and Open Space

The Public Health Service Hospital (PHSH) district is situated on a gentle north-south ridge at the Presidio's southern boundary, overlooking the city and remote from other developed areas of the Presidio. The PHSH evolved as a separate entity, first under the administration of the U.S. Marine Hospital Service and then under the U.S. Public Health Service. The site, originally selected for development in the 1870s because of its proximity to Lobos Creek and Mountain Lake, has been developed into two plateaus, with most of the existing development located on the lower plateau. The district contains 19 buildings, including the former U.S. Marine Hospital and its support buildings. The historic 170,000-square-foot main hospital building, built in 1932, was expanded in 1952 with a seven-story, 128,000-square-foot addition on the south side of the original building. The hospital closed in 1980.

— Maintain the historic concentration of development

on the lower plateau, and enhance open space on the upper plateau.

— Rehabilitate the former hospital for residential use; consider demolition of the non-historic hospital wings, replacing them with more compatible structures.
— Rehabilitate historic housing and accessory structures for a variety of complementary uses.
— Protect and enhance important natural resources, including habitat for rare plant and wildlife species.
— Protect and enhance existing wetland features on the upper plateau.
— Preserve and enhance views to and from the site. Continue and enhance recreational uses.
— Ensure that any new construction is sited and configured to be compatible with the historic district.

The upper plateau behind the hospital supports unique and ecologically significant native plant communities that include coast live oak woodland, central dune scrub, and riparian and dune slack wetland vegetation, as well as the San Francisco lessingia (Lessingia germanorum), a federally-listed endangered plant. The complex array of vegetation also provides valuable habitat for the largest known quail population in San Francisco, as well as other bird species. The potential for historic archeological resources is high in this area. The old Marine Cemetery, a significant archeological resource, dates back to the 1880s.

The PHSH district, historically separate and distinct from the rest of the Presidio's developed areas, will be a setting suitable to residential and educational uses. These building uses may be complemented by compatible outdoor recreational uses. Future planning may consider removal of non-historic structures, including the modern wings of the main hospital building. If a suitable tenant cannot be found to rehabilitate the historic hospital, the entire building may be considered for removal. Removal of the historic hospital and replacement construction would be considered as part of a separate undertaking. The Planning Guidelines would help ensure that any new construction would be sensitive to the prevailing architectural treatment, scale, and orientation of existing structures, and would be designed to reinforce the historic setting. Remnant natural systems in this area will be preserved and revitalized. Ongoing activities in this district include restoration of native plant communities and wildlife corridors, as well as enhancement of the dune slack wetland east of the parking lot below the Nike Missile site. Future projects that might affect the conservation and recovery of the San Francisco lessingia will be carried out in consultation with the U.S. Fish and Wildlife Service.

An Historic Colonial Revival Structure Lends Charm to the Public Health Service Hospital Complex

Access and Circulation

The PHSH building complex has historically been an enclave separate from the rest of the Presidio. Two city streets, 14th and 15th Avenues, provide the main vehicular access. Alternatives for primary access, including reopening the 14th Avenue gate to vehicular access and operating 14th and 15th Avenues as a one-way couplet, will be studied. Access to the PHSH district from other parts of the Presidio will continue along Battery Caulfield Road; through-traffic will be discouraged. Connections to the surrounding network of trails and pathways will provide a scenic pedestrian gateway to other parts of the Presidio. Convenient access will be provided to nearby outdoor recreational amenities such as the Presidio Golf Course, Mountain Lake, and trails.

Planning Guidelines for Public Health Service Hospital District

Spatial Organization and Land Pattern

Upper and Lower Plateaus. Topography has influenced the development of the PHSH site throughout its 125-year history. The building core was sited on a relatively level natural bench in the south-facing slope west of Mountain Lake. An upper plateau above the building core was left more open. This distinction between upper and lower plateaus remains today.

The Public Health Service Hospital District as Seen from Nearby Mountain Lake

Hierarchy of Building Sites

The building complex retains much of the original design of the 1932 plan. Buildings were sited according to function and hierarchy in a campus-like setting. The hospital building retains the most prominent position facing out over the city. Associated buildings are located nearby to the east. Open lawns typically serve as formal foregrounds (front yards) for major buildings or building groups.

Spatial Organisation and Land Paterns Guidelines

— Maintain the historic patterns of development, primarily on the lower plateau. The formal placement of buildings around open spaces and the definition of open space and streets through plantings should be retained. Infill construction should respect historic spatial relationships, scale, and orientation of buildings.

— Enhance open space and preserve natural processes for a functioning ecological system on the upper plateau below the Nike Missile site.

Upper and Lower Pleateaus

Building and Structure

Formal vs. Informal Buildings. The PHSH complex is comprised of the dominant hospital building and a number of smaller buildings. The main institutional structures face the city and present a strong image, with prominent massing and classical detailing. In contrast, the Wyman Avenue houses face east and are arranged in an arc on a knoll, overlooking Mountain Lake and its surroundings. *Contrasting Architectural Character.* The architectural character of the PHSH complex is different from the rest of the Presidio, reflecting its historically separate governmental jurisdiction. The buildings adjoining the hospital structure are organised by function; the use of buff brick and flat red clay tile roofs helps to unify these buildings. Colonial Revival style architecture is used throughout the complex in both institutional and residential structures.

Guidelines for Buildings and Structures

— Maintain the historic character of the site. In concert with historic building rehabilitation, cluster additions and/or replacement construction onto compact sites, close to existing buildings, to reinforce the campus-like setting.

— Ensure that any replacement construction is secondary to the former hospital as the predominant building in the complex.

— Ensure that new construction is compatible in scale, massing, height, color, and materials with the historic buildings in the area. Maximum heights should be between 30 feet to 45 feet for outbuildings and 70 feet for buildings adjacent to the main hospital.

Primary Buildings Clustered on Small Plateau Overlooking City

Open Space/Vegetation/Views

A Rich Mix of Natural Features. The PHSH district is sited on a ridge that drains west to Lobos Creek (the Presidio's source of drinking water) and east to Mountain Lake. Natural areas surrounding the hospital support a variety of native plant habitat, including rare and endangered species. A federally- listed endangered plant species, the San Francisco lessingia, is found on the upper plateau of the site.

Formal Landscaping. Designed landscape features that characterize the PHSH complex include the hospital's front lawn and tree-lined entry roads, the Wyman Street houses' landscapes and tree plantings, the remnant cypress windrow on the north and west sides of the former cemetery, and a large stand of Monterey pine trees north of the hospital.

Site Surrounded by a Diverse Mix of Natural and Cultural Resources

Guidelines for Open Space/Vegetation/Views

- Rehabilitate and restore the upper plateau, below the Nike Missile site, as native plant habitat. Accommodate compatible recreational uses elsewhere consistent with protection of the natural resources.
- Respect the natural and historic terrace landform of the district. Major regrading and construction on slopes should be avoided.
- Protect Lobos Creek, the Presidio's drinking water source, and direct stormwater runoff away from the adjacent watersheds of Lobos Creek and Mountain Lake.
- Consider planting as part of the overall design of the site to articulate and better define historic open spaces and entry sequences.

— Preserve and enhance view corridors and panoramic viewsheds both from and to the site. Significant views include Mountain Lake from Wyman Terrace and Lobos Creek Valley from the western edge of the site, as well as sweeping views of the city and ocean from the upper plateau.
— Restore natural resources, and protect and enhance wetland and endangered species habitat.
— Locate new replacement construction to protect and preserve views and vistas.
— Protect and commemorate the former Marine Cemetery.

Contrast between Formal Orientation of Main Hospital and Informally Sited Adjacent Buildings

Circulation and Access

Access Access Via 14th and 15th Avenues. Historically, a curving, tree-lined drive entered the Presidio at 14th Avenue and ended at the hospital. This access is now gated and provides pedestrian access only. The 15th Avenue gate is the main vehicular entrance to the PHSH district.

Internal Circulation Routes. In the late 1980s, Wedemeyer Street and Battery Caulfield Road were connected to provide access from the PHSH complex to the rest of the Presidio. Circulation within the district is characterized by informal, curving roads that reinforce the site's campus-like character.

Key Trails. Several important trails intersect in the PHSH district. A key section of the Juan Bautista de Anza National Historic Trail runs through the site. The West Pacific Avenue trail extends to Mountain Lake, the Park Boulevard trail connects through the golf course to Washington Boulevard, and the Lobos Creek trail extends through the site to Baker Beach.

Guidelines for Circulations and Access

— Maintain 14th and 15th Avenues as the main access; consider a one-way couplet for vehicles using these streets. A secondary entry should be promoted along Battery Caulfield Road to accommodate traffic coming from within the Presidio.

— Ensure that bike and pedestrian trails connect to the network of nearby local and regional trails.

— Minimize traffic impacts from new uses at the site.

— Enhance public access through improved mass transit options, both within the Presidio and via links to city transit.

HEALTH & SAFETY CODE: CONTINUING CARE FACILITIES

General Provision

Sec. 246.001. SHORT TITLE. This chapter may be cited as the Texas Continuing Care Facility Disclosure and Rehabilitation Act.

Acts 1989, 71st Leg., ch. 678, Sec. 1, eff. Sept. 1, 1989.

Sec. 246.002. DEFINITIONS. In this chapter:

(1) "Board" means the State Board of Insurance.

(2) "Commissioner" means the commissioner of the State Board of Insurance.

(3) "Continuing care" means the furnishing of a living unit, together with personal care services, nursing services, medical services, or other health-related services, regardless of whether the services and the living unit are provided at the same location:

(A) to an individual who is not related by consanguinity or affinity, as determined,

Government Code, to the person furnishing the care; and

(B) under a continuing care contract.

(4) "Continuing care contract" means an agreement that requires the payment of an entrance fee by or on behalf of a resident in exchange for the furnishing of continuing care by a provider and that is effective for:

(A) the life of the resident; or

(B) more than one year.

(5) "Entrance fee" means an initial or deferred transfer of money or other property valued at an amount exceeding three months' rent, made, or promised to be made, as full or partial consideration for acceptance by a provider of a specified individual as a resident. The term does not include a deposit made under a reservation agreement.

(6) "Facility" means a place in which a person provides continuing care to an individual.

(7) "Living unit" means a room, apartment, cottage, or other area that is in a facility and that is set aside for the exclusive use or control of one or more specified individuals.

(8) "Long-term nursing care" means nursing care provided for a period longer than 365 consecutive days.

(9) "Person" means an individual, corporation, association, or partnership, and includes a fraternal or benevolent order or society.

(10) "Provider" means a person who undertakes to provide continuing care in a facility.

(11) "Reservation agreement" means an agreement that requires the payment of a deposit to reserve a living unit for a prospective resident.

(12) "Resident" means an individual entitled to receive continuing care in a facility.

Acts 1989, 71st Leg., ch. 678, Sec. 1, eff. Sept. 1, 1989. Amended by Acts 1991, 72nd Leg., ch. 14, Sec. 95, eff. Sept. 1, 1991; Acts 1991, 72nd Leg., ch. 561, Sec. 31, eff. Aug. 26, 1991; Acts 1993, 73rd Leg., ch. 953, Sec. 1, eff. Sept. 1, 1993; Acts 1995, 74th Leg., ch. 76, Sec. 5.95(27), eff. Sept. 1, 1995.

Sec. 246.003. BOARD POWERS AND DUTIES.

(a) The board shall regulate providers as provided by this chapter.

(b) The board may adopt rules and take other action as necessary to administer and enforce this chapter.

Acts 1989, 71st Leg., ch. 678, Sec. 1, eff. Sept. 1, 1989.

Sec. 246.004. RIGHTS OF RESIDENTS. A resident receiving care in a portion of a facility licensed to provide nursing home care, personal care, or custodial care is entitled to all statutory rights provided to a nursing home, personal care, or custodial care resident.

Acts 1989, 71st Leg., ch. 678, Sec. 1, eff. Sept. 1, 1989.

Sec. 246.005. LICENSING FOR CERTAIN TAX PURPOSES. A facility regulated under this chapter is licensed for purposes of Section 151.314, Tax Code.

Acts 1989, 71st Leg., ch. 678, Sec. 1, eff. Sept. 1, 1989.

Sec. 246.006. QUALITY OF CARE. The commissioner may not regulate or in any manner inquire into the quality of care provided in a facility.

Acts 1989, 71st Leg., ch. 678, Sec. 1, eff. Sept. 1, 1989.

Sec. 246.007. REDUCTION OF FEES. The commissioner shall reduce the annual filing fees under this chapter if the cumulative amount of the fees exceeds the actual cost of regulation.

Acts 1989, 71st Leg., ch. 678, Sec. 1, eff. Sept. 1, 1989.

Certificate of Authority

Sec. 246.021. CERTIFICATE OF AUTHORITY REQUIRED. Unless a provider holds a certificate of authority issued under this subchapter, the provider may not:

(1) acquire a facility;

(2) enter into a continuing care contract; or

(3) enter into a reservation agreement unless the agreement provides for the full refund, for any reason, of a deposit paid in connection with the agreement.

Acts 1989, 71st Leg., ch. 678, Sec. 1, eff. Sept. 1, 1989. Amended by Acts 1993, 73rd Leg., ch. 953, Sec. 2, eff. Sept. 1, 1993.

Sec. 246.022. APPLICATION FOR AND ISSUANCE OF CERTIFICATE OF AUTHORITY.

(a) The commissioner shall adopt rules stating the information an applicant for a certificate of authority must submit.

(b) On receiving an application for a certificate of authority, the commissioner shall conduct a hearing on the application.

(c) The commissioner shall grant an application for a certificate of authority if the commissioner finds that:

(1) the applicant or the facility is financially sound;

(2) the competence, experience, and integrity of the applicant, its board of directors, its officers, or its management make it in the public interest to issue the certificate; and

(3) the applicant is capable of complying with this chapter.

(d) The commissioner shall issue an order approving or disapproving an application not later than the 180th day after the date on which the application is filed.

(e) The commissioner may limit issuance of certificates of authority to incorporated entities only.

Acts 1989, 71st Leg., ch. 678, Sec. 1, eff. Sept. 1, 1989.

Sec. 246.023. MANDATORY ISSUANCE OF CERTIFICATE OF AUTHORITY TO CERTAIN FACILITIES.

(a) The commissioner shall issue a certificate of authority for a facility that:

(1) was occupied by at least one resident on September 1, 1987;

(2) was under construction on September 1, 1987; or

(3) incurred substantial financial obligations before September 1, 1987, related to the development of the facility.

(b) A certificate of authority issued under this section may be suspended or revoked as any other certificate.

(c) This section prevails over Section 246.022.

Acts 1989, 71st Leg., ch. 678, Sec. 1, eff. Sept. 1, 1989.

Sec. 246.024. TRANSFER OF CERTIFICATE OF AUTHORITY. A certificate of authority may not be transferred without the prior approval of the commissioner.

Acts 1989, 71st Leg., ch. 678, Sec. 1, eff. Sept. 1, 1989. Amended by Acts 1991, 72nd Leg., ch. 14, Sec. 96, eff. Sept. 1, 1991.

Sec. 246.025. SUSPENSION OR REVOCATION OF CERTIFICATE OF AUTHORITY.

The commissioner may suspend or revoke a provider's certificate of authority if the provider:

(1) draws on its entrance fee escrow in an amount greater than provided for by Section 246.073;

(2) draws on its loan reserve fund escrow in an amount greater than provided for by Section 246.078; or

(3) intentionally violates this chapter.

Acts 1989, 71st Leg., ch. 678, Sec. 1, eff. Sept. 1, 1989. Amended by Acts 1991, 72nd Leg., ch. 14, Sec. 97, eff. Sept. 1, 1991.

Sec. 246.026. MANAGEMENT BY OTHERS. A holder of a certificate of authority may not contract for management of the facility unless the commissioner is notified of the contract.

Acts 1989, 71st Leg., ch. 678, Sec. 1, eff. Sept. 1, 1989.

Sec. 246.027. CERTIFICATE OF AUTHORITY FEES.

(a) Except as provided by Subsection (b), a facility that files an application for a certificate of authority must pay to the commissioner a fee of $10,000.

(b) A facility that files an application for a certificate of authority issued under Section 246.023 must pay to the commissioner:

(1) a fee of $500; and

(2) a fee of $2 for each living unit in the facility, excluding a unit devoted to that portion of the facility that is a licensed nursing home.

Acts 1989, 71st Leg., ch. 678, Sec. 1, eff. Sept. 1, 1989.

Continuing Care Contracts and Disclosure Statements

Sec. 246.041. PRECONTRACTUAL RECORDING REQUIREMENTS.

(a) A provider shall file with the board a current disclosure statement that meets the requirements of this subchapter and shall file copies of the agreements establishing the escrows under Subchapter D or a verified statement explaining that an escrow is not required before the provider:

(1) contracts to provide continuing care in a facility located or to be located in this state;

(2) extends the term of an existing continuing care contract in a facility that is located or to be located in this state and that requires or allows an entrance fee from any person, regardless of whether the extended contract requires an entrance fee; or

(3) including a person acting on the provider's behalf, solicits for an individual who is a resident of this state a continuing care contract in this state.

(b) A contract is solicited in this state if, during the 12-month period preceding the date on which a continuing care contract for a facility is signed or accepted by either party, information concerning the facility or the availability of a continuing care contract for the facility is given:

(1) by personal, telephone, mail, or other communication directed to and received by a person at a location in this state; or

(2) in a paid advertisement published or broadcast from within this state, other than in a publication

in which more than two-thirds of the circulation is outside this state.

Acts 1989, 71st Leg., ch. 678, Sec. 1, eff. Sept. 1, 1989.

Sec. 246.042. DELIVERY OF DISCLOSURE STATEMENT.

(a) A provider who has not been issued a certificate of authority under Subchapter B must deliver a disclosure statement to any person from whom the provider accepts a deposit in connection with a reservation agreement before the provider accepts the deposit.

(b) A provider who has been issued a certificate of authority under Subchapter B must deliver a disclosure statement to a person with whom a continuing care contract is to be made before the earlier of:

(1) the execution of the continuing care contract; or

(2) the transfer of any entrance fee or nonrefundable deposit to the provider by or on behalf of the person.

(c) The most recently filed disclosure statement is the only statement that:

(1) is current for purposes of this chapter; and

(2) may be delivered under this section.

Acts 1989, 71st Leg., ch. 678, Sec. 1, eff. Sept. 1, 1989. Amended by Acts 1993, 73rd Leg., ch. 953, Sec. 3, eff. Sept. 1, 1993.

Sec. 246.043. COVER PAGE OF DISCLOSURE STATEMENT.

The cover page of a disclosure statement must state:

(1) the date of the statement in a prominent location and in type that is boldfaced, capitalized, underlined, or otherwise set out from the surrounding written material so as to be conspicuous;

(2) that if the provider has not been issued a certificate of authority under Subchapter B, this chapter requires the delivery of a disclosure statement to a prospective resident before the payment of any deposit to reserve a living unit;

(3) that this chapter requires the delivery of a disclosure statement to a contracting party before the execution of a continuing care contract or the payment of an entrance fee or nonrefundable deposit; and

(4) that the disclosure statement has not been approved by a governmental agency or representative to ensure the accuracy of its information.

Acts 1989, 71st Leg., ch. 678, Sec. 1, eff. Sept. 1, 1989. Amended by Acts 1991, 72nd Leg., ch. 14, Sec. 98, eff. Sept. 1, 1991; Acts 1993, 73rd Leg., ch. 953, Sec. 4, eff. Sept. 1, 1993.

Sec. 246.044. CONTENTS OF DISCLOSURE STATEMENT: PROVIDER.

(a) The disclosure statement must include the name and business address of the provider and a statement of whether the provider is a partnership, corporation, or other type of legal entity. If the provider is not an individual, the statement must include:

(1) the name and business address of each officer, director, trustee, and managing or general partner; and

(2) the name and business address of each person who has at least a 10 percent interest in the provider and a description of the person's interest in or occupation with the provider.

(b) The provider may include in the disclosure statement any other material information concerning the facility or the provider.

Acts 1989, 71st Leg., ch. 678, Sec. 1, eff. Sept. 1, 1989.

Sec. 246.045. CONTENTS OF DISCLOSURE STATEMENT: THIRD PARTY MANAGEMENT.

If a person, other than an individual directly employed by the provider, is to be the day-to-day manager of a facility, the disclosure statement must include:

(1) a description of the person's business experience, if any, in the operation or management of a similar facility;

(2) the name and address of any professional service, firm, association, trust, partnership, or corporation that:

(A) has in the person, or in which the person has, at least a 10 percent interest; and

(B) proposes to provide goods, leases, or services to the facility or to the residents of the facility, of an aggregate value of at least $500 in a year;

(3) a description of any goods, leases, or services under Subdivision (2), and a statement of their probable or anticipated cost to the facility, provider, or residents, or a statement that their cost cannot be estimated; and

(4) a description of any matter in which the person:

(A) has been convicted of a felony, pleaded nolo

contendere to a felony charge, or has been held liable or enjoined in a civil action by final judgment, if the felony or civil action involved fraud, embezzlement, fraudulent conversion, or misappropriation of property;

(B) is subject to an injunction or restrictive order of a court of record; or

(C) has had any state or federal license or permit suspended or revoked as a result of an action brought by a governmental agency if the order or action arose out of or was related to a business activity in a health care field, including an action affecting a license to operate a foster care facility, a nursing home, a retirement home, a home for the aged, or a facility subject to this chapter or a similar statute in another state.

Acts 1989, 71st Leg., ch. 678, Sec. 1, eff. Sept. 1, 1989.

Sec. 246.046. CONTENTS OF DISCLOSURE STATEMENT: AFFILIATION WITH NONPROFIT ORGANIZATION.

The disclosure statement must state whether the provider is affiliated with a religious, charitable, or other nonprofit organization, and if so, the statement must:

(1) describe the extent of the affiliation;

(2) explain the extent to which the organization is responsible for the financial and contractual obligations of the provider; and

(3) cite any provision of the Internal Revenue Code of 1986 under which the provider or affiliate claims to be exempt from the payment of income tax.

Acts 1989, 71st Leg., ch. 678, Sec. 1, eff. Sept. 1, 1989.

Sec. 246.047. CONTENTS OF DISCLOSURE STATEMENT: PHYSICAL PROPERTY.

(a) The disclosure statement must provide the location and a description of the proposed or existing physical property of the facility.

(b) If the physical property of the facility is proposed, the disclosure statement must state:

(1) the estimated completion date;

(2) whether construction has begun; and

(3) any contingencies under which construction may be deferred.

Acts 1989, 71st Leg., ch. 678, Sec. 1, eff. Sept. 1, 1989.

Sec. 246.048. CONTENTS OF DISCLOSURE STATEMENT: CONTRACTS AND FEES. The disclosure statement must describe:

(1) the services provided at the facility under a continuing care contract, including:

(A) the extent to which medical care is furnished; and

(B) those services that are included for specified basic fees for continuing care and those services that are made available at extra charge;

(2) all fees required of residents, including the entrance fee and any periodic charges;

(3) the conditions under which a continuing care contract at the facility may be canceled by the provider or the resident;

(4) any conditions under which all or part of the entrance fee is refundable on cancellation of the contract by

the provider or the resident, or by the death of the resident before or during the occupancy of a living unit; and

(5) the manner by which the provider may adjust periodic charges or other recurring fees and any limitations on those adjustments.

Acts 1989, 71st Leg., ch. 678, Sec. 1, eff. Sept. 1, 1989.

Sec. 246.049. CONTENTS OF DISCLOSURE STATEMENT: CHANGE OF CIRCUMSTANCES. The disclosure statement must state:

(1) the policy of the facility regarding changes in the number of people residing in a living unit because of marriage or other relationships;

(2) the policy of the facility relating to the admission of a spouse to the facility and the consequences if the spouse does not meet the requirements for admission;

(3) the conditions under which a living unit occupied by a resident may be made available by the facility to a different resident other than on the death of the previous resident; and

(4) the health and financial conditions required for acceptance as a resident and for continuation as a resident, including the effect of any change in the health or financial condition of an individual between the date of the continuing care contract and the date on which the individual initially occupies a living unit.

Acts 1989, 71st Leg., ch. 678, Sec. 1, eff. Sept. 1, 1989.

Sec. 246.050. CONTENTS OF DISCLOSURE STATEMENT: FINANCIAL INFORMATION.

(a) The disclosure statement must:

(1) describe any provisions made or to be made to provide reserve funding or security to enable the provider to fully perform its obligations under a continuing care contract at a facility, including:

(A) the establishment of escrow accounts, trusts, or reserve funds and the manner in which those funds will be invested; and

(B) the name and experience of any individual in the direct employment of the provider who will make the investment decisions; and

(2) provide financial statements of the provider, including:

(A) a balance sheet as of the end of the most recent fiscal year; and

(B) income statements and a statement of cash flow for each of the three most recent fiscal years that the provider has been in existence.

(b) Financial statements required by Subsection (a)(2) must be prepared in accordance with generally accepted accounting principles and must be audited by an independent certified public accountant, who shall state in the audit report whether the financial statements were prepared in accordance with those principles.

Acts 1989, 71st Leg., ch. 678, Sec. 1, eff. Sept. 1, 1989. Amended by Acts 1991, 72nd Leg., ch. 14, Sec. 99, eff. Sept. 1, 1991.

Sec. 246.051. CONTENTS OF DISCLOSURE STATEMENT: ANNUAL INCOME STATEMENTS. The disclosure statement must contain estimated annual income statements for the facility for at least five fiscal years, including:

(1) anticipated earning on any cash reserves;

(2) estimates of net receipts from entrance fees, other than entrance fees included in the statement of anticipated source and application of funds required under Section 246.052, minus estimated entrance fee refunds, including a description of the actuarial basis and method of computation for the projection of entrance fee receipts;

(3) an estimate of gifts or bequests to be relied on to meet operating expenses;

(4) a projection of estimated income from fees and charges, excluding entrance fees, that:

  (A) states individual rates anticipated to be charged; and

  (B) includes a description of the assumptions used for computing the estimated occupancy rate of the facility and the effect on the income of the facility of any government subsidies for health care services to be provided under the continuing care contract;

(5) a projection of the facility's operating expenses, including:

  (A) a description of the assumptions used in computing the expenses; and

  (B) a separate allowance for the replacement of equipment and furnishings and anticipated major structural repairs or additions; and

(6) an estimate of annual payments of principal and interest required by a mortgage loan or other long-term financing arrangement relating to the facility.

Acts 1989, 71st Leg., ch. 678, Sec. 1, eff. Sept. 1, 1989. Amended by Acts 1991, 72nd Leg., ch. 14, Sec. 100, eff. Sept. 1, 1991.

Sec. 246.052. CONTENTS OF DISCLOSURE STATEMENT: ANTICIPATED SOURCE AND APPLICATION OF FUNDS. If a facility has not begun operation, the disclosure statement must include a statement of the anticipated source and application of the funds to be used in the purchase or construction of the facility, including:

(1) an estimate of the cost of purchasing or constructing and of equipping the facility, including financing expenses, legal expenses, land costs, occupancy development costs, and similar costs that the provider expects to incur or to become obligated to pay before operations begin;

(2) a description of any mortgage loan or other long-term financing arrangement for the facility, including the anticipated terms and costs of the financing;

(3) an estimate of the total entrance fees to be received from, or on behalf of, residents before the operation of the facility begins; and

(4) an estimate of any funds anticipated to be necessary to cover initial losses and to provide reserve funds to assure full performance of the obligations of the provider under a continuing care contract.

Acts 1989, 71st Leg., ch. 678, Sec. 1, eff. Sept. 1, 1989.

Sec. 246.053. STANDARD CONTRACT FORM.

(a) A copy of the standard contract form used by a provider must be attached as an exhibit to each disclosure statement.

(b) The standard contract form must specify the refund provisions of Sections 246.056 and 246.057.

Acts 1989, 71st Leg., ch. 678, Sec. 1, eff. Sept. 1, 1989. Amended by Acts 1991, 72nd Leg., ch. 14, Sec. 101, eff. Sept. 1, 1991.

Sec. 246.054. ANNUAL DISCLOSURE STATEMENT REVISION.

(a) A provider shall file a revised disclosure statement with the board not later than the 120th day after the date on which the provider's fiscal year ends.

(b) The revised disclosure statement must revise, as of the end of the provider's fiscal year, the information required by this subchapter.

(c) The revised disclosure statement must describe any material differences between:

(1) the estimated income statements filed under Section 246.052 as a part of the disclosure statement filed after the start of the provider's most recently completed fiscal year; and

(2) the actual result of operations during that fiscal year with the revised estimated income statements filed as a part of the revised disclosure statement.

(d) A provider may revise its disclosure statement and may file the revised disclosure statement at any other time if, in the provider's opinion, revision is necessary to prevent a disclosure statement from containing a material misstatement of fact or omitting a material fact required to be included in the disclosure statement.

(e) The commissioner shall review the disclosure statement for completeness but is not required to review the disclosure statement for accuracy.

Acts 1989, 71st Leg., ch. 678, Sec. 1, eff. Sept. 1, 1989.

Sec. 246.055. ADVERTISEMENT IN CONFLICT WITH DISCLOSURES. A provider may not engage in any type of advertisement for a continuing care contract or facility if the advertisement contains a statement or representation in conflict with the disclosures required under this subchapter.

Acts 1989, 71st Leg., ch. 678, Sec. 1, eff. Sept. 1, 1989.

Sec. 246.056. RESCISSION OF CONTRACT; REQUIRED LANGUAGE.

(a) A person who executes a continuing care contract with a provider may rescind the contract at any time before the later of midnight of the seventh day, or a later day if specified in the contract:

(1) after the date on which the continuing care contract is executed; or

(2) after the date on which the person receives a disclosure statement that meets the requirements of this subchapter.

(b) A resident who executes a continuing care contract may not be required to move into the facility before the expiration of the period during which the contract may be rescinded.

(c) If a continuing care contract is rescinded under this section, any money or property transferred to the provider, other than periodic charges specified in the contract and applicable only to the period a living unit was actually occupied by the resident, shall be refunded not later than the 30th day after the date of rescission.

(d) Each continuing care contract must include the following statement or a substantially equivalent statement in type that is boldfaced, capitalized, underlined, or otherwise set out from the surrounding written material so as to be conspicuous: "You may cancel this contract at any time prior to midnight of the seventh day, or a later day if specified in the contract, after the date on which you sign this contract or you receive the facility's disclosure statement, whichever occurs later. If you elect to cancel the contract, you must do so by written notice and you will be entitled to receive a refund of all assets transferred other than periodic charges applicable to your occupancy of a living unit."

(e) Each continuing contract also must include the following statement in type that is boldfaced, capitalized, underlined, or otherwise set out from the surrounding written material so as to be conspicuous: "This document, if executed, constitutes a legal and binding contract between you and _____. You may wish to consult a legal or financial advisor before signing, although it is not required that you do so to make this contract binding."

Acts 1989, 71st Leg., ch. 678, Sec. 1, eff. Sept. 1, 1989. Amended by Acts 1991, 72nd Leg., ch. 14, Sec. 102, eff. Sept. 1, 1991; Acts 1993, 73rd Leg., ch. 953, Sec. 5, eff. Sept. 1, 1993.

Sec. 246.057. CANCELLATION OF CONTRACT: DEATH OR INCAPACITY BEFORE OCCUPANCY.

(a) A continuing care contract is canceled if the resident:

(1) dies before occupying a living unit in the facility; or

(2) is precluded under the terms of the contract from occupying a living unit in the facility because of illness, injury, or incapacity.

(b) If a continuing care contract is canceled under this section, the resident or the resident's legal representative is entitled to a refund of all money or property transferred to the provider, minus:

(1) any nonstandard costs specifically incurred by the provider or facility at the request of the resident that are described in the contract or in an addendum to the contract signed by the resident; and

(2) a reasonable service charge, if set out in the contract, that may not exceed the greater of $1,000 or two per cent of the entrance fee.

Acts 1989, 71st Leg., ch. 678, Sec. 1, eff. Sept. 1, 1989. Amended by Acts 1993, 73rd Leg., ch. 953, Sec. 6, eff. Sept. 1, 1993.

Sec. 246.058. DISCLOSURE STATEMENT FEES.

A facility that files a disclosure statement under Section 246.041 or 246.054 shall pay to the commissioner:

(1) a filing fee of $500; and

(2) a fee of not more than $2 for each living unit in the facility, excluding a unit devoted to that portion of the facility that is a licensed nursing home.

Entrance Fee and Reserve Fund Escow Accounts

Sec. 246.071. ENTRANCE FEE ESCROW ACCOUNT; ESCROW AGENT.

(a) Before a provider may accept the payment of a deposit made under a reservation agreement or any portion of an entrance fee, the provider must establish an entrance fee escrow account with a bank or trust company, as escrow agent, that is located in this state.

(b) The provider shall deposit with the escrow agent any deposit or any portion of an entrance fee received by the provider not later than 72 hours after the provider receives the deposit or fee.

Acts 1989, 71st Leg., ch. 678, Sec. 1, eff. Sept. 1, 1989. Amended by Acts 1993, 73rd Leg., ch. 953, Sec. 7, eff. Sept. 1, 1993.

Sec. 246.072. RETURN OF DEPOSITS; RELEASE OR RETURN OF ENTRANCE FEE.

(a) On a written request from or on behalf of the provider or a prospective resident, the escrow agent shall return the amount on deposit to the person who paid the deposit or shall maintain the deposit as an entrance fee in the entrance fee escrow account.

(b) Unless the escrow agent receives a written request from or on behalf of a provider or a resident for the return of an entrance fee under Section 246.056, the agent shall release the fee to the provider or place the fee in a loan reserve fund escrow.

Acts 1989, 71st Leg., ch. 678, Sec. 1, eff. Sept. 1, 1989. Amended by Acts 1991, 72nd Leg., ch. 14, Sec. 104, eff. Sept. 1, 1991; Acts 1993, 73rd Leg., ch. 953, Sec. 8, eff. Sept. 1, 1993.

Sec. 246.073. RELEASE TO THE PROVIDER.

(a) Except as provided by Subsection (b), an escrow agent shall release an entrance fee to the provider if:

(1) a minimum of 50 percent of the number of living units in the facility have been reserved for residents, as evidenced by:

(A) uncanceled executed continuing care contracts with those residents; and

(B) the receipt by the agent of entrance fee deposits of at least 10 percent of the entrance fee designated in each continuing care contract;

(2) the total amount of aggregate entrance fees received or receivable by the provider under binding continuing care contracts, the anticipated proceeds of any first mortgage loan or other long-term financing commitment described under Subdivision (3), and funds from other sources in the actual possession of the provider are equal to or more than the total amount of:

(A) 90 percent of the aggregate cost of constructing or purchasing, equipping, and furnishing the facility;

(B) 90 percent of the funds estimated, in the statement of anticipated source and application of funds included in the disclosure statement, to be necessary to cover initial losses of the facility; and

(C) 90 percent of the amount of any loan reserve fund escrow required to be maintained by the provider under Section 246.077; and

(3) a commitment has been received by the provider for any permanent mortgage loan or other long-term financing described in the statement of anticipated source and application of funds included in the current disclosure statement and any conditions of the commitment before disbursement of funds have been substantially satisfied, other than completion of the construction or closing on the purchase of the facility; and:

(A) if construction of the facility has not been substantially completed:

(i) all necessary government permits or approvals have been obtained;

(ii) the provider and the general contractor responsible for construction of the facility have entered into a maximum price contract;

(iii) a recognized surety authorized to do business in this state has executed in favor of the provider a bond covering faithful performance of the construction contract by the general contractor and the payment of all obligations under the contract;

(iv) the provider has entered a loan agreement for an interim construction loan in an amount that, when combined with the amount of entrance fees in escrow plus the amount of funds from other sources in the actual possession of the provider, equals or exceeds the estimated cost of constructing, equipping, and furnishing the facility;

(v) the lender has disbursed not less than 10 percent of the amount of the construction loan for physical construction or completed site preparation work; and

(vi) the provider has placed orders at firm prices for not less than 50 percent of the value of items necessary for equipping and furnishing the facility in accordance with the description in the disclosure statement, including any installation charges; or

(B) if construction or purchase of the facility has been substantially completed:

(i) an occupancy permit covering the living unit has been issued by the local government that has authority to issue the permit; and

(ii) if the entrance fee applies to a living unit that has been previously occupied, the living unit is available for occupancy by the new resident.

(b) Before the date on which the loan reserve fund escrow required under Section 246.077 is first established, the aggregate amount of entrance fees that may be released to the provider under this section may not exceed an amount equal to the aggregate amount of entrance fees received or receivable by the provider under binding continuing care contracts minus the amount of entrance fees received or receivable that are required to be maintained initially in the loan reserve fund escrow.

Acts 1989, 71st Leg., ch. 678, Sec. 1, eff. Sept. 1, 1989. Amended by Acts 1991, 72nd Leg., ch. 14, Sec. 105, eff. Sept. 1, 1991; Acts 1993, 73rd Leg., ch. 953, Sec. 9, eff. Sept. 1, 1993.

Sec. 246.074. RETURN OF ENTRANCE FEE.

The escrow agent shall return an entrance fee to the person who paid it if the fee is not released to the provider or placed in the loan reserve fund escrow required under Section 246.077 within:

(1) 36 months after the date on which any portion of the entrance fee is received by the provider; or

(2) a longer time specified by the provider in the disclosure statement delivered with the continuing care contract under which the fee was paid.

Acts 1989, 71st Leg., ch. 678, Sec. 1, eff. Sept. 1, 1989. Amended by Acts 1991, 72nd Leg., ch. 14, Sec. 106, eff. Sept. 1, 1991; Acts 1993, 73rd Leg., ch. 953, Sec. 10, eff. Sept. 1, 1993.

Sec. 246.075. ESCROW OF APPLICATION FEE NOT REQUIRED.

This subchapter does not require the escrow of any nonrefundable portion of a deposit or entrance fee that:

(1) does not exceed an amount equal to two percent of the entrance fee; and

(2) is clearly designated as nonrefundable in the continuing care contract or reservation agreement.

Acts 1989, 71st Leg., ch. 678, Sec. 1, eff. Sept. 1, 1989. Amended by Acts 1993, 73rd Leg., ch. 953, Sec. 11, eff. Sept. 1, 1993.

Sec. 246.076. INTEREST ACCRUED ON ENTRANCE FEE FUNDS.

Unless otherwise provided in a continuing care contract, interest that accrues on funds held in an entrance fee escrow account is the property of the provider.

Acts 1989, 71st Leg., ch. 678, Sec. 1, eff. Sept. 1, 1989. Amended by Acts 1993, 73rd Leg., ch. 953, Sec. 12, eff. Sept. 1, 1993.

Sec. 246.077. RESERVE FUND ESCROW.

(a) When a facility is first occupied by a resident, the provider shall establish and maintain in an escrow account with a bank or trust company, as escrow agent, that is located in this state a reserve fund equal to the total of all principal and interest payments due during the next 12 months on any first mortgage loan or other long-term financing arrangement for the facility. The requirements of this section may be met in whole or in part by other reserve funds held for the purpose of meeting loan obligations if the total amount equals or exceeds the amount required by this subsection.

(b) At the option of the facility, the loan reserve fund escrow amount may exclude the portion of principal and interest payments applicable to that portion of the facility that is a licensed nursing home.

(c) The provider shall maintain the loan reserve fund escrow in an account that is fully covered by federal deposit insurance and is separate from the provider's business account or in other accounts or investments approved by the commissioner. The funds in the reserve fund escrow account may be invested, with earnings payable to the provider.

Acts 1989, 71st Leg., ch. 678, Sec. 1, eff. Sept. 1, 1989. Amended by Acts 1991, 72nd Leg., ch. 14, Sec. 107, eff. Sept. 1, 1991.

Sec. 246.078. RELEASE OF RESERVE FUND ESCROW.

(a) The escrow agent may release an amount equal to not more than one-twelfth of the loan reserve fund required by Section 246.077 if the provider requests the release in writing.

(b) The escrow agent must give written notice to the board not later than the 11th day before the date of the release.

(c) The escrow agent may not release funds from the loan reserve fund escrow under this section more than once during a calendar year. A provider at any time may apply to the commissioner for the withdrawal of all or part of the loan reserve escrow funds. The provider may withdraw the funds on the approval of the withdrawal by the commissioner. The application must be made and the approval given as provided by rule.

(d) The provider must repay to the loan reserve fund escrow account the amount released to the provider under Subsection (a) or (c) not later than 18 months after the date the amount is released. The commissioner may place the provider or facility under supervision under Section 246.091 or take any other appropriate action as provided by law if the provider does not repay the loan reserve fund escrow account within the required period.

Acts 1989, 71st Leg., ch. 678, Sec. 1, eff. Sept. 1, 1989. Amended by Acts 1991, 72nd Leg., ch. 14, Sec. 108, eff. Sept. 1, 1991.

Sec. 246.079. TRANSITION.

(a) A provider who operates a facility that existed on September 1, 1987, must comply with the filing requirements imposed under Section 246.041 and the escrow requirements imposed under Sections 246.077 and 246.078 not later than September 1, 1990.

(b) The commissioner may extend the time for compliance under this section for a reasonable period if the commissioner determines that the provider is unable to comply with this section after making a good faith effort to comply.

Acts 1989, 71st Leg., ch. 678, Sec. 1, eff. Sept. 1, 1989. Amended by Acts 1991, 72nd Leg., ch. 14, Sec. 109, eff. Sept. 1, 1991.

Sec. 246.080. APPLICABILITY. Sections 246.071 through 246.076 do not apply to a facility that on September 1, 1987, was completed and occupied by at least one person.

Added by Acts 1991, 72nd Leg., ch. 14, Sec. 110, eff. Sept. 1, 1991.

Supervision, Rehabilitation, and Liquidation

Sec. 246.091. SUPERVISION BY COMMISSIONER.

(a) The commissioner may place a provider or facility under supervision if:

(1) the provider draws on the provider's entrance fee escrow in an amount greater than permitted by Section 246.073;

(2) the provider draws on the provider's loan reserve fund escrow in an amount greater than permitted or more frequently than permitted by Section 246.078;

(3) the commissioner determines, after a complaint and investigation, that the provider is financially unsound or is unable to meet the income or available cash projections previously filed by the provider and that the ability of the provider to fully perform its obligations under continuing care contracts is endangered; or

(4) the provider is bankrupt, insolvent, or has filed for protection from creditors under a federal or state reorganization, bankruptcy, or insolvency law.

(b) The commissioner appoints the supervisor.

(c) The commissioner may provide that the provider may not, during the supervision period and without the prior approval of the commissioner or the supervisor:

(1) dispose of, convey, or encumber its assets;

(2) withdraw its bank accounts;

(3) lend its funds;

(4) invest its funds;

(5) transfer its property;

(6) incur a debt, obligation, or liability; or

(7) merge or consolidate with another facility.

(d) The commissioner shall terminate the supervision and restore to a provider the authority to manage the affairs of the facility if the commissioner determines that the facility is capable of meeting its financial obligations.

(e) The facility or provider shall pay the costs of a supervisor.

Acts 1989, 71st Leg., ch. 678, Sec. 1, eff. Sept. 1, 1989. Amended by Acts 1991, 72nd Leg., ch. 14, Sec. 111, eff. Sept. 1, 1991.

Sec. 246.092. APPLICATION FOR COURT ORDER FOR REHABILITATION OR LIQUIDATION.

(a) The commissioner shall request the attorney general to apply to a district court of this state, or to the federal bankruptcy court that has exercised jurisdiction over a provider or facility, for an order directing the appointment of a trustee to rehabilitate or liquidate the facility if the commissioner elects not to place the facility under supervision and:

(1) the provider draws from the provider's loan reserve fund escrow an amount greater than permitted by Section 246.078;

(2) the provider does not repay the loan reserve fund escrow as required by Section 246.078;

(3) the board determines, after a complaint and investigation, that the provider is financially unsound or is unable to meet the income or available cash projections previously filed by the provider and that the ability of the provider to fully perform its obligations under continuing care contracts is endangered; or

(4) the provider is bankrupt, insolvent, or has filed for protection from creditors under a federal or state reorganization, bankruptcy, or insolvency law.

(b) In connection with an application for an order to rehabilitate or liquidate a facility, the court shall consider the manner in which the welfare of persons who have previously contracted with the provider for continuing care at the facility may be best served, and may order that the proceeds of a lien imposed under Section 246.111 may be used in full or partial payment of entrance fees to other facilities on behalf of the residents of the facility being liquidated.

Acts 1989, 71st Leg., ch. 678, Sec. 1, eff. Sept. 1, 1989. Amended by Acts 1991, 72nd Leg., ch. 14, Sec. 112, eff. Sept. 1, 1991.

Sec. 246.093. ORDER TO REHABILITATE. An order to rehabilitate a facility must direct the trustee to:

(1) take possession of the provider's property in order to conduct the business, including employing any managers or agents the trustee considers necessary; and

(2) take action as directed by the court to eliminate the causes and conditions that made rehabilitation necessary.

Acts 1989, 71st Leg., ch. 678, Sec. 1, eff. Sept. 1, 1989.

Sec. 246.094. ORDER TO LIQUIDATE.

(a) If the trustee determines that further efforts to rehabilitate the provider would be impractical or useless, the trustee may apply to the court that ordered the rehabilitation for an order of liquidation.

(b) A court that has jurisdiction may issue an order to liquidate a facility on application of the board, regardless of whether an order to rehabilitate the facility exists. If the court issues an order to liquidate, the court shall appoint a trustee to collect and liquidate all of the provider's assets located in this state.

(c) A person may not contract for continuing care at a facility after an order to liquidate that facility has been entered.

Acts 1989, 71st Leg., ch. 678, Sec. 1, eff. Sept. 1, 1989.

Sec. 246.095. BOND. A court may refuse to make or may vacate an order to rehabilitate under this subchapter if the provider posts a bond that is:

(1) in an amount determined by the court to be equal to the reserve funding needed to fulfill the provider's obligations under its continuing care contracts at the facility;

(2) issued by a recognized surety authorized to do business in this state; and

(3) executed in favor of the state on behalf of all persons entitled to refunds of entrance fees from the provider or other damages if the provider is unable to fulfill its continuing care contracts at the facility.

Acts 1989, 71st Leg., ch. 678, Sec. 1, eff. Sept. 1, 1989.

Sec. 246.096. TERMINATION OF REHABILITATION.

(a) A court may terminate a rehabilitation and order return of a facility and its assets and affairs to the management of the provider if the court, on petition of the trustee or the provider or on its own motion, finds that:

  (1) the objectives of the order to rehabilitate the facility have been accomplished; and

  (2) the facility can be returned to the provider's management without further jeopardy to the

residents, creditors, or owners of the facility or the public.

(b) A court may enter an order under this section after:

(1) a full report and accounting of the conduct of the facility's affairs during the rehabilitation; and

(2) a report on the facility's financial condition.

Acts 1989, 71st Leg., ch. 678, Sec. 1, eff. Sept. 1, 1989.

Sec. 246.097. PAYMENT OF TRUSTEE. The reasonable costs, expenses, and fees of the trustee are payable from the assets of the facility.

Enforcement

Sec. 246.111. LIEN.

(a) To secure the obligations of the provider under any continuing care contract, a lien attaches on the date a resident first occupies a facility. The lien covers the real and personal property of the provider located at the facility. The provider shall prepare a written notice sworn to by an officer of the provider for each county where the provider has a facility. The notice must contain the name of the provider, the legal description of each facility of the provider, and a statement that the facility is subject to this chapter and the lien provided by this section. The provider shall file for record the notice in the real property records of each county where the provider has a facility on or before the later of January 1, 1994, or the date of the execution of the first continuing care contract relating to the facility.

(b) The commissioner may remove a lien under this section if requested by a provider to obtain secondary financing or refinancing of a facility if:

(1) the facility is financially sound; and

(2) removal of the lien does not adversely affect the residents.

(c) A lien under this section is subordinate to any liens on the property of the facility if the proceeds of the loan secured by the liens were used in whole or in part to:

(1) construct, acquire, replace, or improve the facility; or

(2) refinance an earlier loan used to construct, acquire, replace, or improve the facility.

(d) A lien under this section is effective for 10 years.

(e) A lien under this section may be foreclosed on application of the board if the facility is liquidated or the provider is insolvent or bankrupt. The proceeds from a foreclosed lien shall be used for full or partial satisfaction of the provider's obligations under continuing care contracts in effect on the date of the foreclosure.

Acts 1989, 71st Leg., ch. 678, Sec. 1, eff. Sept. 1, 1989. Amended by Acts 1993, 73rd Leg., ch. 953, Sec. 13, 15, eff. Sept. 1, 1993.

Sec. 246.112. INVESTIGATIONS. The commissioner may conduct an examination or investigation as necessary to:

(1) determine whether a person has violated or is about to violate this chapter;

(2) aid in the enforcement of this chapter;

(3) determine the financial solvency of a facility; or

(4) verify a statement contained in a disclosure statement filed or delivered under this chapter.

Acts 1989, 71st Leg., ch. 678, Sec. 1, eff. Sept. 1, 1989.

Sec. 246.113. PRODUCTION OF EVIDENCE.

(a) In an investigation or proceeding under this chapter, the board may:

(1) require or allow a person to file a written statement regarding any of the facts and circumstances concerning the matter to be investigated;

(2) administer oaths and affirmations;

(3) subpoena witnesses;

(4) compel attendance;

(5) take evidence; and

(6) require the production of any books, papers, correspondence, memoranda, agreements, or other documents or records considered relevant to the inquiry.

(b) The board may bring suit in district court to enforce a subpoena if the person to whom a subpoena is directed fails to comply.

Acts 1989, 71st Leg., ch. 678, Sec. 1, eff. Sept. 1, 1989.

Sec. 246.114. ACTUARIAL REVIEW.

(a) This section applies only to a facility whose contracts offer future guarantees of long-term nursing care that develop current actuarial liabilities.

(b) A facility subject to this section that initially filed with the commissioner an actuarial review performed on or after September 1, 1982, and before September 1, 1987, shall file with the commissioner subsequent actuarial reviews at five-year intervals from the date of completion of the initial actuarial review.

(c) A facility subject to this section that initially filed with the commissioner an actuarial review performed on or after September 1, 1987, shall file with the commissioner subsequent actuarial reviews at five-year intervals from the date of the filing of the initial actuarial review.

(d) The commissioner may require an actuarial review of a facility before the end of the five-year interval in which the facility would otherwise be required to file an actuarial review if, in the opinion of the commissioner, the facility exhibits conditions of financial instability warranting an earlier review.

Acts 1989, 71st Leg., ch. 678, Sec. 1, eff. Sept. 1, 1989. Amended by Acts 1991, 72nd Leg., ch. 14, Sec. 113, eff. Sept. 1, 1991; Acts 1993, 73rd Leg., ch. 953, Sec. 14, eff. Sept. 1, 1993.

Sec. 246.115. CEASE AND DESIST ORDERS; INJUNCTIONS.

(a) The board may request that the attorney general bring an action to prohibit a person from engaging in an act or practice and to order compliance with this chapter if the board determines, after a complaint or by other means, that the act or practice violates this chapter or an order made under this chapter.

(b) The action may be brought in the district court of a county in which:

(1) the defendant resides;

(2) the defendant has done business;

(3) the principal place of business of the defendant is located; or

(4) the transaction occurred.

(c) The court may grant an injunction or restraining

order on a proper showing. If the court grants an injunction or restraining order, the court shall issue it without bond.

Acts 1989, 71st Leg., ch. 678, Sec. 1, eff. Sept. 1, 1989.

Sec. 246.116. CRIMINAL PENALTY.

(a) A person commits an offense if the person intentionally violates this chapter.

(b) An offense under this section is a Class A misdemeanor.

Acts 1989, 71st Leg., ch. 678, Sec. 1, eff. Sept. 1, 1989.

Sec. 246.117. CIVIL LIABILITY.

(a) A provider who makes a continuing care contract without complying with the disclosure statement requirement under Subchapter C, or who makes a continuing care contract with a person who has relied on a disclosure statement that omits a material fact required to be stated in the statement or necessary to make the statement accurate, is liable to the person with whom the continuing care contract is made for:

(1) actual damages;

(2) repayment of all fees paid to the provider minus the reasonable value of care and lodging provided to the person by or on whose behalf the continuing care contract was made before the violation, misstatement, or omission was discovered or reasonably should have been discovered;

(3) interest at the legal rate for judgments;

(4) court costs; and

(5) reasonable attorney's fees.

(b) A provider is liable under this section regardless of whether the provider had actual knowledge of the misstatement or omission.

(c) A person may not file or maintain an action under this section if the person, before filing the action, received a written offer of a refund of all amounts paid to the provider, facility, or person violating this chapter and reasonable interest from the date of payment, minus the reasonable value of care and lodging provided before the receipt of the offer and:

   (1) the offer states the provisions of this section; and

   (2) the recipient of the offer fails to accept the offer within 30 days after the date the offer is received.

(d) A person must bring suit under this section not later than three years after:

   (1) the date on which the continuing care contract was entered into; or

   (2) the violation, misstatement, or omission is discovered or reasonably should have been discovered.

(e) Except as expressly provided by this chapter, civil liability does not arise in favor of a private party by implication from or as a result of the violation of this chapter or a rule or order adopted under this chapter.

(f) This chapter does not limit a liability that would exist under any other statute or common law if this chapter were not in effect.

(g) The provisions of this chapter are not exclusive and the remedies provided by this chapter are in addition to any other remedies provided by any other law.

THE BATTLE TO MAKE HEALTH CARE WORK

Do HMOs Serve Only HMOs?

Will a system set up to maximise profit ever truly care for patients? One indication comes from looking at how HMOs organise their lists of approved drugs, or formularies, for their doctors to use. As one might expect, the drugs are often the cheapest and typically not the best. For instance, PacifiCare, now the nation's largest HMO for Medicare recipients, replaced an effective, high-cost schizophrenia drug called Risperdal with the low-cost, 36 year-old drug, Haldol. A thirty-day supply of Risperdal costs $240 compared to $2.50 for a similar supply of Haldol — nearly a 1,000% savings for PacifiCare. But the side effects of the inferior Haldol include severe, uncontrollable shaking. While such penuriousness at the expense of patients has come to be expected from HMOs, the example of how Foundation Health considered organising its formulary shows that the hunt for profits never ends. Sabin Russell, a veteran health care writer at the *San Francisco Chronicle*, exposed a proposal by Bristol-Myers Squibb that would have given Foundation Health a million dollars a month as a fee for restricting its formulary exclusively to the products of the drug maker.

"The draft agreement calls for Bristol-Myers to pay $1 million per month, for up to three years, to Sacramento-based Integrated Pharmaceutical Services," Russell reported, meaning a total fee of $36 million. "A Foundation Health subsidiary, IPS is a 'pharmacy benefits management' company that handles drug benefits of more than four million HMO members across the country. The deal appears to be the latest twist on a little-known practice called rebating, in which drug companies pay cash to insurers, hospitals and even doctor groups for high-volume sales of their products."

The rub with this kick-back was that the drugs in question were *neither* the most cost-effective nor medically effective in the class of drugs. Still, "preferred" status on the HMO drug list would go to Bristol-Myers' blood pressure drugs Monopril and Avapro; the antibiotic Cefzil; Plavix, a drug that inhibits blood clotting; and cholesterol-lowering drug Pravachol. Patients who wanted or needed other drugs, which are more effective or less costly, would have to circumnavigate a time-consuming appeals process. Foundation Health simply considered the deal for its $1 million per month kick-back at the expense of patients and the medical system. According to Russell, "In fact, the Bristol-Myers draft agreement appears to rule out passing the payments to consumers. The drug company 'contribution' the memo states, 'is not an additional discount...and is not intended for benefit of payor organisations whose pharmacy benefits are managed by IPS.'"

Another troubling aspect of the arrangement, as the *Chronicle's* Russell reports, is who makes the choices about which drugs Health Net would cover. Once the choices were in the hands of a committee of the HMO's participating doctors. Now, acting on the advice of a new committee of hired consultants, the choices are made by Health Net executives. This kind of profit-at-all-costs orientation is having an impact, even on those in industry. "Along the hallways at Sprint headquarters here [in Kansas City, Missouri], the great expectations for managed care have dimmed," reported the *New York Times* in October 1998. "In a score of interviews with workers and managers, no one recounted the kind of HMO horror story that makes headlines: the wrong leg amputated, a child denied a transplant. Instead, they said they had found managed care to be exasperating, callous and sometimes just senseless." Health care executives and large employers both admit that quality has been a casualty of the managed care system. Amazingly, an academic survey of health care industry executives found that almost half — 49% — believe the growth of managed care has *decreased* the quality of patient care. (At the same time, not surprisingly, 55% say there is no need for increased federal regulation of HMOs; 52% believe there is no need for more state regulation.)

Employers concur. In 1998, 42% of employers polled believed cost pressures are hurting the quality of care, up from 33% in 1997 and 28% in 1996.

Small employers are particularly disturbed, despite the pro-HMO leanings of the National Federation of Independent Business (NFIB). In a June 1998 Kaiser Family Foundation/ Harvard survey of 800 executives of small businesses conducted for the American Small Business Alliance, 66% of the executives support enacting a new law to allow patients to sue their HMO as a way to make sure people get the care they need, rather than oppose it as unnecessary government intrusion.

Managing costs does not mean the proper management of treatment. As we have seen in too many cases, those goals are often antagonistic. Moreover, corporations managing their own money well does not translate to the health care system managing its costs effectively. Columbia's multi-billion dollar bilking of the taxpayer is one clear example. The recent HMO industry practice of dumping elders, because the companies are no longer permitted to cherry pick only the healthy seniors in Medicare, is another. In mundane ways, too, HMO corporations have incentives and opportunities to make money for themselves at the expense of both cost-effectiveness and health-enhancement of the health care system.

"The price one pays to keep health care affordable is a degree of aggravation," Health Net chief medical officer Dr. Alan Zwerner told Russell. But affordable for whom? The company or the provision of a reasonable standard of health care? Americans are learning from the growing exposure to HMO medicine that a system set up to manage money will never truly take care of patients. HMO corporations will simply shift costs away from themselves. The public and the patient will pay. HMO corporations will continue to charge. But what alternatives do we have?

Big "R" Reforms

The HMO reform debate has taken place in state legislatures and Congress. In the province of politicians, the process has lent itself mostly to sound and fury without progress. Efforts to maintain a firewall between money managers and healers have fallen victim to the entrenched HMO lobby.

"They killed the health care Patients' Bill of Rights," Vice President Gore said at a White House press conference in October 1998. "I was in — I was in John Dingell's district in Dearborn — and this is a true story — an emergency room doctor told us of a man who came in to the emergency room in full cardiac arrest, his heart stopped, the doctor eventually brought him back to life. The HMO refused to pay the bill and said it was not an emergency. The man was dead! (Laughter.)"

The *New York Times* reported in October 1998 that consumers' complaints about health insurers and HMOs are "surging," according to state health insurance commissioners. Interviews with twelve state insurance departments in the most densely populated states show that health care complaints have grown "50% over the last one to three years, far faster than the growth of enrollment in managed care plans." Audiences across the nation cheered when the lead actress denounced HMOs in the 1997 movie, "As Good As It Gets."

During 1998, politicians in Congress and state legislatures, however, failed to enact many serious reforms, folding under pressure from the HMO lobby. The Patients' Bill of Rights was defeated in Congress. The Republicans offered fig-leaf reforms with no enforceable remedies. The insurance industry is similarly attempting to prevent states from regulating managed care plans. In July 1999, the Republican-controlled United States Senate passed purported patient rights legislation that did not include significant reforms. The G.O.P. plan allegedly applied to 48 million Americans in federally regulated health plans, but in fact only 10% of that population are actually enrolled in HMOs. Vice President Al Gore said the minimal measure would be vetoed because, "it's a fraud." Senior G.O.P. Senator John Chaffee (Rhode Island) told the Associated Press, "What have we accomplished? It seems to me we've let down the American people." In the debate over curbing HMO power, everyone — from patient advocates, to doctors, to the HMO industry — has his own definition of "reform." The HMO industry favours greater disclosure and a so-called external review system, where patients' disputes with their HMO are appealed to a third party for review rather than heard before a court or jury.

Those on the side of the patient — consumer groups, nurses, doctors — have made the right-to-sue without ERISA's hurdles the litmus test for genuine HMO reform. In 1998, the American Medical Association, which for decades supported capping the damages of doctors and hospitals for medical negligence, shunned its sacred cow of national damage limits. GOP leaders offered this carrot to the AMA in an attempt to split the ERISA-reform coalition, but in a valiant act, the AMA refused to take it. Real reform must stem from serious accountability measures. Can we get there? Can we create and regulate a system that puts public health first, so that the many tragedies told in this book never appear again in our wealthy country?

One vital step is the distinction between three types of reforms, each of which will be considered in turn. "First tier" reforms would even the playing field for patients, so that they have the necessary leverage over their HMOs to get the care they need and deserve. "Second tier" changes, discussed later, would fundamentally alter the health care system to provide coverage to more patients at less cost. Lastly, it is crucial to see through the third tier of phony reforms and political placebos the HMO industry has put forth in order to stave off genuine, systemic correctives.

Level-The-Playing-Field Reforms — Nailing Down Tier One

Restore the right to sue for damages at the federal level. The most "ripe" reform for those who know the system is to apply the same liability laws to HMOs now faced by every other industry in America. As discussed, federal ERISA law shields HMOs that administer private employer-paid insurance from damages for wrongdoing, so there is never a price to pay in court.. Congress can and should amend ERISA. Damages should be available under state common law when HMOs that administer employer-paid health care commit fraud, negligence, are responsible for a wrongful death, or breach the covenant of good faith and fair dealing that applies to every other type of business. From 1974 until 1987, patients with employer-paid benefits could receive damages against insurers. With the 1987 *Pilot Life v. Dedeaux* ruling, state common law was preempted in a way that the federal framers of ERISA did not intend. The easiest way to close the ERISA loophole is for Congress to specifically clarify the province of state courts and juries over HMOs that administer benefits. The Congressional Budget Office reported in July 1998 that giving patients the right to sue would add no more than 1.2% to health care premiums, including the costs of so-called defensive medicine. At the time of this publication, in July 1999, a bipartisan "compromise" in Congress would give patients the right to recover only compensatory damages, such as lost wages, not punitive damages, which punish wrongdoing.

Unless HMOs face significant damages, they will continue to ignore patients' needs and doctors' recommendations. In most states patients cannot collect for their pain and suffering after their death, so HMOs could have an incentive to actually let them die without punitive damages.

States can enact new HMO liability laws to protect against profiteering HMOs that put money ahead of good medicine. States can pass legislation that specifically skirts the ERISA loophole and hold HMOs accountable for their decisions by creating a new "corporate negligence" cause of action for HMOs. HMOs do deny treatment, overturn doctors' decisions and dictate limits on medical treatments and care. New state laws could require that HMOs be held accountable for reckless health care decisions. As noted, Texas recently became the first state in the nation to offer its citizens a way around ERISA to protect themselves against poor quality medical care. The Texas law assures that the physician, not the HMO, is in charge of patient care. This begins to restore the doctor-patient relationship. HMOs are liable when they exercise "influence or control which result in the failure to exercise ordinary care," in other words accountable for medical negligence and quality-of-care issues.

In the fall of 1998, a federal district court judge upheld

the Texas statute because, "In this case, the Act addresses the quality of benefits actually provided. ERISA 'simply says nothing about the quality of benefits received.' Dukes, 57 F.3d at 3576." By contrast, the Court struck down the Texas independent review process as preempted by ERISA, because it deals with determinations of coverage disputes. The review process is the HMO industry's alternative to liability. California legislators are also considering another way around ERISA. Pending legislation makes use of a clause in ERISA that "saves" for the states the right to regulate the business of insurance. The bill specifically makes damages available under the state's insurance law when HMOs breach their insurance contracts. If the legislation passes, HMOs will no doubt sue to invalidate it.

Creation of an independent non-profit consumer watchdog association funded by voluntary contributions, and governed by a board with a majority elected by members. For years, utility consumers in three states have been able to unite in order to fight fraud and unnecessarily high rates because of Consumer Utility Boards or CUBs. These voluntary associations have been effective because they have been able to contact every utility ratepayer in the state and ask them to voluntarily join. The key to this reform — devised by consumer advocate Ralph Nader — is a voluntary "check off" on the utility bill, which allows consumers to join the association with a minimal contribution ($5–$12 per year).

Congress, the state legislature, or the people via ballot initiative in some states can establish a similar consumer association (a public corporation) for patients in HMOs. It could be granted access to insurance company mailing lists and the power to advocate on behalf of individuals or groups of patients, and to publish reports on quality-of-service provided by HMOs, hospitals, nursing homes, and other health care businesses. The association would be a check on the health care industry's business practices, working to ensure that the profit motive does not diminish the standard of care and invade the doctor-patient relationship. An effective consumer health care organisation could save lives. Already CUBs have saved consumers billions of dollars. The Illinois Citizens Utility Board, with 200,000 members, has saved Illinois taxpayers more than $3 billion since 1983 by challenging utility rate hikes, and has successfully educated ratepayers on how to save money on services and on conservation issues. This vehicle is a model for HMO patients to join together to increase accountability and standards of care. It would be a democratic organisation of HMO members interested solely in quality medical care.

Prohibit mandatory and secret arbitration of medical grievances as a condition for health coverage. As previously noted, most HMOs and managed care plans *require* the consumer to give up his rights to go to court in cases of malpractice or in disputes over quality of care — *as a condition of coverage*. Instead of having access to the public forum of a court, patients are forced into a system of mandatory binding arbitration. Forced arbitration is costly, unfair, and conceals quality-of-care violations from public scrutiny. Many states now prohibit mandatory binding arbitration agreements. Arizona's constitution, for instance, specifically bars any legislative limitation on the right to trial. However, in too many states, forced arbitration enables HMOs to hide from juries and judges in a secret and often biased justice system. Reforms to end binding arbitration as a condition of health coverage would force HMOs that delay and deny care to face the scrutiny of an open courtroom. This would publicly air quality-of-care violations so that they are not repeated.

Require prior approval from regulators before HMOs and insurers can raise their premiums or lower the rates they pay doctors via capitation. The property/casualty insurance industry has a system in most states in the nation requiring state approval before rates are raised or lowered, as opposed to the old "file and use" system, where the insurers simply filed the rate and used it. No such system is in place for health insurance, despite its life and death stakes. As mentioned earlier, many individual policyholders with Blue Cross of California saw their rates skyrocket by 58% in 1998. Elderly Kaiser individual members in Washington, D.C. saw a 49.4% increase in premiums. Older Americans can become costly patients and the HMOs hope to discourage them from staying. HMOs say that the young should not subsidize the old, but this is precisely the definition of an insurance pool risk. You pay in when you are young and healthy, and utilize when you are older and sicker. Requiring prior approval for rate increases, and an opportunity for a public hearing and comment, will keep the HMO industry honest. Utilities face this scrutiny, and health care is certainly as vital a public commodity as water and power.

Health care businesses should be required to show the need for rate increases and where and how the money would be used. A fair rate of return must be set on health care companies and HMOs. If care is to be rationed, so should HMO profits. HMOs have used their leverage to squeeze down the capitated rates for doctors so low that it is virtually impossible for physicians to do all they can for their patients. Some primary care doctors receive rates as low as $6 dollars per month for all the care of a patient. A prior approval system could require that HMOs show that the capitated rates paid to their physicians and medical groups are actuarially sound and sufficient to take care of the patients' needs — particularly the sickest patients. If the rates paid to physicians who treat a disproportionate number of sick patients are not "risk adjusted" upward, doctors will simply compete for well patients. The public has a compelling interest in this type of rate regulation to make sure the insurance system serves the sick as well as the healthy.

Ban full-risk capitation. The idea of pitting doctors' financial interests against their patients' quality of care violates the fundamental doctor-patient relationship. Today some doctors accept nearly full risk for all of a patient's care, meaning almost *all* costs expended on the patient are paid by the doctors, not the HMO. This development happened without public debate, comment or approval. Large physician medical groups act essentially like insurers, without the solvency requirements to make sure they are fiscally secure or hold an insurance company license. Whatever doctors spend on patients comes out of their own pockets. "The less you do for patients, the more money you make" is an unacceptable public policy for most Americans. The federal government can outlaw the payment of capitated rates to physicians, or at least "full risk" capitated payments that turn physicians into insurers. If HMOs are prevented from passing full risk, or even any risk, on to physicians, then the fire wall between the doctor's focus on care and business concerns will be rebuilt.

Prohibiting HMO bureaucrats from second-guessing physicians who examine patients. HMOs claim that if they can no longer capitate doctors, they will have to increase the number and interference of company bureaucrats. An HMO should not be allowed to deny a patient a physician-recommended treatment unless another equally qualified doctor has examined the patient and made a medical determination that the care is not warranted. In addition, any HMO employee making treatment decisions should have a valid medical license in that state.

Would the HMO industry really oppose such basic reforms? Yes. In 1997 and 1998, California's HMO industry fought such legislation twice. The reform, aimed at curtailing the overriding of doctors' decisions, focused on extreme cases, where a patient's life and health was certified to be in jeopardy by the first doctor who examined them. The industry prevailed on Governor Pete Wilson to veto this eminently reasonable reform. This common sense rule of law, however, must be applied to HMOs if bureaucrats are to be prevented from overruling qualified doctors and making life and death decisions. In particular, if capitation is prohibited, this reform will ensure that HMO bureaucrats do not interfere in the doctor-patient relationship when a doctor is seeking critical care for his patients. This vital legislation returns control over medicine to doctors, not accountants.

States must set safe staffing standards so that nurses and doctors are available to patients based on acuity of illness, regardless of whether the patient is in a nursing home or in a hospital. Typically, staffing protections exist only for the most severely ill patients in critical care units. Even in these areas, some businesses routinely violate the law. Stronger penalties are needed. Safe staffing requirements do not currently exist for hospital units outside of critical care, nursing homes, medical offices, and same-day surgery centers. This is why HMOs often seek to shunt patients who need to be in the hospital to so-called skilled nursing facilities or nursing homes, which are less costly because doctors and nurses do not have to be on the premises in any ratio to the patient population. Until safe nurse- and physician-staffing levels are set by regulators for all acute patients, HMOs and insurers will continue to cut corners and strand patients in inappropriate settings based solely on cost.

Mandate public disclosure of data on health care quality, financial information and complaints and arbitrations against the health care organisation. One of the key components of our medical system should be informed consent by patients. HMOs may deal with questions of life or death, but they are under no obligation to tell you anything about their day-to-day operations. They do not disclose how they determine whether you receive needed care, how much money they make based on those decisions or about why any legal actions were taken against them. HMOs should be required to publicly disclose all information relating to quality of patient care. This includes all data and studies used to determine quality, staffing, and reduction of services; financial reports, including corporate affiliates or subsidiaries; and complaints and arbitrations. Today HMOs claim they are trying to get more information into consumers' hands. But this information is often useless. For instance, patient-satisfaction surveys are often taken among people who are well and rarely use their HMO. And private report cards are maintained by industry-sponsored groups such as the Joint Commission on the Accreditation of Healthcare Organisations (JCAHO) and National Committee For Quality Assurance (NCQA).

NCQA was formed in 1979 by the trade associations for the managed care industry — the American Managed Care and Review Association and the Group Health Association of America. The group was founded, in fact, to counter the federal government's attempts to monitor HMOs. The main funding source for NCQA continues to be HMOs, although the group is seeking to diversify its funding to appear more independent. In 1997, NCQA's board of directors was a "Who's Who" of HMO executives and corporate chieftains, including representatives from Aetna, Blue Cross, Henry Ford Health System, PacifiCare, Harvard Pilgrim Health Care. NCQA has created its own performance measurements, the Health Plan Employer Data & Information Set (HEDIS). "The critical point here is that 'value' as used by NCQA is to be measured strictly in terms of *cost* of health care delivery, as distinguished from the clinical needs of a patient as defined by the trained professional," said former U.S. Justice Department attorney Kenneth Anderson, an expert in anti-trust law who contends NCQA is a part of collusive behaviour among the managed care industry. "Thus, the NCQA criteria by which performance is measured are initially framed by those entities — HMOs, managed care companies and employer payers — who have a strong incentive to define 'appropriate' levels of care in narrow economic (e.g. cost) terms."

Anderson says "This NCQA effort is, in part, essentially a massive public relations programme orchestrated by the managed care industry in hopes of averting the establishment of a truly independent and objective mechanism, whether private or governmental, to define what quality health care really is and then measure plan performance against such standards." As for JCAHO, a July 1996 audit by the national consumer group Public Citizen found JCAHO "views hospitals not as entities to be regulated, but as customers to be serviced and kept satisfied." Part of the basis for the finding is that twenty-one out of twenty-eight members of the JCAHO's Board of Commissioners were industry representatives who each paid $20,000 a year for a seat.

Prohibit health care businesses from selling medical records without the express written authorisation of the patient. Here is a scary thought: It is easier for people to find out if you have cancer or AIDS than it is for them to get a list of the videos you have rented. Patient records are now a commodity for sale.

Hospitals, HMOs, and drug companies all maintain commercial data banks which collect and store individual medical records, containing sensitive personal information. Most states' civil codes have extensive provisions for maintaining medical confidentiality, but most were written before the computer explosion. The new technology changes everything and leaves patients extremely vulnerable. Dr. Beverly Woodward, an ethicist at Brandeis University, says employees at most Boston-area hospitals enter patient information directly on-line without consent from the patient. Any doctor at any affiliated hospital can access these records, including psychiatric records. In Maryland, Medicaid clerks tapped into computers and accessed critical patient information — names, addresses, incomes, medical records — which they sold, sometimes for less than fifty cents per head, to HMO recruiters. Breach of privacy can have serious consequences. Patients with AIDS or mental illnesses have a great deal to lose if their condition is made public — sometimes their jobs, even their families.

Prohibit HMOs, hospitals, nursing homes or other health care businesses from firing, delisting or retaliating against doctors and licensed caregivers who speak out on behalf of patients or who report patient care violations to authorities. "Gag" or "disparagement" clauses in contracts between physicians and HMOs or insurers pressure doctors to keep silent about practices or policies they believe may be injurious to patients. Hospitals have fired, sanctioned, and threatened doctors, nurses and other licensed caregivers who advocate for their patients, challenge unsafe practices or cooperate with official investigations. These pernicious practices must be barred if doctors are to be trusted by their patients.

HMOs say "gag" clauses do not exist today. If they do not, there is no reason not to ban them.

Fixing Long-term Care Insurance — Integrating Support Systems. The average life expectancy has lengthened more in the last 100 years than in the previous 2,000. People are living longer, but their final years are not necessarily healthier. Half of all women and a third of all men 65 years of age and older will spend their last years in a nursing home, at a cost of about $40,000 a year.

Long-term care is the assistance people need when they are not able to accomplish some of the basic "activities of daily living" like bathing, dressing, walking or moving from the bed to a chair. The National Center for Health Care Statistics reported in 1996 that half of those 85 and older require long-term care assistance. Unfortunately, traditional health insurance and Medicare will generally not cover home care or community-assisted nursing home living. One must be poor or become poor before becoming eligible for long-term care benefits through Medicaid. Standard health policies pay less than 1% of long term care costs. Medicare covers less than 4%. Private payments, which are costly to individuals and their families, account for 29%. Medicaid — which covers the poor and those who have "spent-down" their assets (a difficult process) — accounts for 68% of the payments. Should it take becoming poor or disabled, or driving your family into poverty, in order to qualify for home-care coverage? Shut-ins who cannot afford home care develop bed sores or anorexia, then need to be hospitalized at a much higher cost.

Long-term care in California averages about $124 a day, or about $45,000 a year. According to the Brookings Institute only 4 to 5% of the elderly nationwide have some kind of private long-term care coverage. Marketing is not prompting consumers to buy policies at a younger age — the average purchaser of private long-term care insurance is 68 years-old. Plus, policies are sold almost exclusively on an individual, rather than group, basis, with concomitant high administrative costs for insurers. According to the National Association of Insurance Commissioners (NAIC), annual premiums for long-term care insurance can run as much as $2,000 for the average-aged purchaser. Premiums increase as one gets older and there are so many options in policies that even sophisticated consumers have difficulty understanding what they are buying and how it compares with other products.

Deceptive and fraudulent marketing is also increasingly a serious problem for long-term care insurance. federal legislation in 1996 created a national long-term care insurance policy to be sold by private insurers. Drafted at the behest of the insurance industry, the federal policy provides less generous benefit payments than many state-based policies, including California's — eliminating the most common form of disability, the inability to walk, as a trigger for paying benefits. The insurance lobby sold the less generous benefits policy to Congress, and then marketed it to seniors, under the pretense that because the policy's cost was tax deductible, older Americans would benefit. The problem is that the vast majority of seniors do not itemize their medical deductions and will not reap a tax benefit.

The affordability and availability of long-term care must be addressed in a coherent national health care policy, particularly as it relates to Medicare and Medicaid. Can society afford to pay to keep all older Americans alive as long as they and their family want and technology allows? Critical to answering this question is a more reasonable long-term care public policy. One solution is for the federal government to issue long-term care insurance that includes the most common form of disability — the inability to walk — and for it to be jointly underwritten by private companies. A second potential solution is to build long term care insurance into the federal Medicare package, so that families will not have to "spend-down" or "go-bankrupt" just to get nursing home care. Surveys show that the majority of the American public agree with expanding Medicare to include long term care. Private companies like Columbia/HCA have milked and bilked the homecare market at the expense of the taxpayer, mostly through Medicaid. Meanwhile, those doing the job are underpaid and overworked. Integrating the continuum of home care into the medical care delivery system is vital to cost-effectiveness and health enhancement.

Systemic Changes: The Second Tier Reforms

Important as they are, first-tier reforms will not fundamentally alter the drive to sacrifice care in the name of profit. More potent, systemic remedies like those enumerated below are likely needed.

End For-Profit, Investor Ownership of HMOs and Health Care Businesses. Medical care is not a commodity. It should not be bought and sold like automobiles. Health care does not fit the logic of the market. Many observers trace the reckless, profit-driven care-cutting at HMOs and managed care companies to the rise of for-profit, investor-owned HMOs and health care businesses. The easy money in managed care, though, is long gone. How do investor-owned HMOs respond to the current serious slide in their stock? They move to fewer facilities, reduced access to specialists, cheaper drugs, shorter hospital stays, fewer doctors and hospitals, less caution. In the current environment, the maintenance of the company's rate of return to attract investors demands that patients pay the price. The HMO network of doctors is made more restrictive, research and training programmes are cut, doctors are fired.

Former United States Surgeon General C. Everett Koop and John Baldwin, the dean of the medical school at Dartmouth College, posed the question of control of health care this way: "Sustained profits require aggressive cost-cutting. This results, inevitably, in restriction of access and withholding of care. But do we really want to relegate such decisions to analysts within the health care industry, or should we assert the public interest in these crucial ethical, societal and medical issues?"

When California-based PacifiCare bought failing FHP International in 1997, for instance, the executives and directors took home millions. FHP patients had already paid the price. Long before the sale, about one-third of FHP doctors were fired, training programmes were dismantled and the drug list cut, according to FHP's founder, in order to dress the company up for sale by clearing FHP's books of expensive overhead. FHP shareholders, who took the HMO officers to court, claimed unscrupulous board members and executives purposely destroyed a viable and healthy company just to sell off its resources and make millions for themselves. Without new controls to protect health resources, the current system is clearly open to raids by profiteers. In the $9 billion U.S. Healthcare merger with Aetna in 1996, for instance, U.S. Healthcare chief Leonard Abramson walked away with over $900 million. PacifiCare medical directors, who are responsible for approving or denying physician requests for expensive drugs and treatment, view a constantly updated electronic ticker-tape of the company's stock price on the wall above the elevator to their offices. These medical directors decide physician requests that could affect that stock price. Do business or medical decisions rule?

Patients deserve a moratorium on for-profit HMO takeovers of not-for- profit HMOs, hospitals and clinics. This would discourage the quick buck mentality by HMO executives while protecting the availability and accessibility of health care. Medical resources are far too valuable a public commodity to evaporate the next time a Wall Street bubble bursts. A ban on for-profit, investor ownership of HMOs would put HMOs back in the hands of doctors and health care professionals who have been trained to run the system.

A study in the July 14, 1999 edition of the *Journal of the American Medical Association* found that not-for-profit HMOs deliver a better quality of care than investor-owned, for-profit HMOs in fourteen categories selected by the NCQA. For instance, investor-owned HMOs had lower rates of immunisation, mammography and psychiatric hospitalisation. One can only imagine how much better still the non-profits would perform if they did not have to compete in markets dominated by for-profit companies. Some might say that doctors are for-profit enterprises themselves. This is correct. But, unlike HMOs, physicians also hold medical licenses that can be taken away and they can be held accountable in a court of law in every state. Effective checks on physician conflict of interest can be maintained. Doctors working within the framework of a non-profit medical system will have additional ethical constraints. HMOs are starting to fail financially. Oxford in New York, for instance, fell apart after its stock tumbled. New Jersey officials were forced to take over HIP Health Plans of New Jersey in October of 1998 because it was bordering on insolvency. Governor Christine Whitman's administration announced that it wants to create a safety net for patients by exploring the possibility of a "guaranty fund" for HMOs — which, unlike traditional insurers, do not have reserve requirements. The stress on HMO finances will only continue.

For-profit HMOs operate in a climate of profiteering and investor demands for a strong rate of return on their capital. The non-profit HMOs compete in the same environment as the for-profits — trying to undercut their for-profit competitors' prices. This is what happened to Kaiser, a non-profit, competing in a for-profit environment. Kaiser reduced its once excellent service to maintain its price levels for employers. A disillusioned Paul Ellwood, the father of HMOs, who even coined the term managed care, relayed recently, "A Kaiser official told me the other day, 'Until better quality attracts more patients, I don't care about it any more. We've been talking about quality improvement for thirty or forty years without much to show for it.'" The non-profits are subject to the same downsizing demands to lower costs in order to cut premiums so they can attract more customers. Take the investor-owned, for-profit company out of the managed care equation and the management of quality care within a budget will be the primary concern, rather than return on investment. The non-profit medical group can return to its primary goal of treating patients.

Boycott HMOs and Receive Health Care Direct From Employers. Motorola Corporation received so many complaints from its employees about their HMOs that it created a new system where the company itself contracts with a network of doctors and hospitals to take care of its employees' medical needs. Motorola cut out the unnecessary middle men — the HMOs and insurance companies. Employees report greater satisfaction with their health care and doctors say they now are the ones in control of managing care, knowing they must contain costs (or they will lose their contracts), but not at the expense of medically necessary treatment. Motorola's vice president for benefits, Rick Dorozil, told CBS News, "We will continue to do this as long as we can do it faster, better, cheaper, and at better quality." For $12.50 a week and 10% of bills, employees and their families can see any doctor in the network, including specialists, without preauthorisation. Seventy percent of Motorola's 80,000 employees have enrolled in this new plan. As more employers follow suit in this voluntary arrangement, at least patients with employer-paid health care will have more options. There are two daunting problems with this model. First, employers have access to personal medical information about their employees. This creates a very real threat to patient privacy. AIDS patients, for instance, might find themselves out of work and filing discrimination lawsuits because of a bigoted employer. Most obviously, those without employer-paid health care would still have to deal with HMOs, and these patients would tend to be seniors on Medicare, the disabled and poor on Medicaid, and others without jobs or with low-paying jobs — people who tend to be sicker. HMOs would have to serve a sicker population without taking in the premiums from the healthier working population. This system would be destined to collapse. HMO medicine, which prefers to take in dollars from the healthy and limit care for the sick, would be destroyed by adverse selection — the "risk pool" being drained of the best risks and left with the worst. A more comprehensive national strategy is warranted precisely because we must have one health care system that shares the risk equally for the healthy and the sick rather than many systems which compete for the healthiest and leave the sickest to the taxpayer's generosity.

The Fox Guarding the Henhouse: Avoiding HMO Attempts to Control Reform

Privatisation advocates have long tried to turn public control of our schools, courts, public assistance systems and municipal services over to private corporations in the name of greater efficiency. But Aetna, PacifiCare, Kaiser and others among the nation's largest HMOs have actually tried to privatize legislative reforms of their own industry by promising to implement private "independent" review systems, where the HMO voluntarily pays a third party to review patient problems, rather than submit to public mandates.

State and federal legislators cannot trust the HMO industry's promise to reform itself. The HMOs' independent review systems purport to give patients facing delays and denials an appeal, but deliver infrequently.

First, reviewing companies are hardly 'independent' of the HMOs that contract and pay for their services. For instance, marketing communications from one such company, Medical Care Management Corporation of Bethesda Maryland, to HMO clients boast that the company "can save payers millions of dollars a year on just a few cases. Our expert physicians affirm the high cost, high risk procedures submitted for review in one-half to two-thirds of cases, depending on the type of disease and the patient's profile. If you are paying for 100 such cases now, inadvisable treatments may be costing you over $6 million." So the so-called independent reviewers market a "denial" rate of 33–50%.

California actually already enacted an "independent" review system in 1996 for patients in need of "experimental procedures" when standard therapies do not work. In theory, this "independent" review system was unassailable, but in practice no reviewing agency was accredited for six months to perform reviews under the law. Subsequently only two were accredited, one of which was Medical Care Management Corporation. Other companies have been unable or unwilling to prove their "independence" through detailed disclosure about their financial ties to HMOs, their protocols and their reviewers.

Appeals decided by such companies are the HMO industry's reform of choice because the private process permits bureaucratic maneuvers by HMOs against which the seriously ill patient has neither the time nor capacity to defend. Folsom, California resident Barbara Brown, once a teacher of the year, ran up against this situation when she contracted advanced ovarian cancer and standard treatments would not do. On July 1, 1998 she appealed under California's new experimental treatment law. With no accredited reviewers, Kaiser picked an agency of its choice, Medical Care Management Corporation. Barbara says, "First, Kaiser made every effort to control all the information that went into the review process...Second, Kaiser biased the panel of experts against my proposed experimental therapy by steering the experts toward Kaiser's own leading set of questions...Third, in their reports, the experts all stated that their assigned role was to respond to Kaiser's questions."

Denied life-saving treatment by both Kaiser's internal grievance process and then its so-called external review, Barbara was forced to sell her house to pay for her treatment. Only a community bake sale and car wash that raised $25,000 provided the down payment for her care. Barbara is now recovering. Her "experimental" surgery, which her HMO said would kill her, resulted in the complete removal of all visible tumor from her abdomen. As of this writing in June 1999, she has had ten healthy months with her family. However, creditors are still pursuing her and she has had to move out of her home.

Private review systems are no substitute for civic scrutiny. Congress and state legislatures must not be deterred from enacting right-to-sue legislation and other public mandates. The wealthiest nation on earth must impose its civil values on private corporations rather than let the fate of mothers like Barbara Brown depend on the success of car washes and bake sales. Third-party reviewing systems will only work well in conjunction with public laws for HMO accountability. Companies must know that if they do not play fair they will face large damage awards or other fines. Texas's independent review process, for instance, has been held out as successful, but the state is the only in the nation where a patient can take an HMO to state court for quality-of-care violations. The independent review and liability laws were passed simultaneously. While the review process was struck down by a federal judge as in violation of ERISA, the state and HMOs reached a voluntary agreement to continue using the system. A private system of appeal without ultimate public accountability is destined to betray the HMO patient. Legislators who forget their public mandate to reform HMOs and favour a private solution do their constituents a grave disservice.

The Final Frontier: The Uninsured

National Preventive Health Care

One of HMO medicine's biggest promises was to reduce the number of uninsured Americans by making insurance more affordable. Unfortunately, HMO medicine has failed on this front too. The Census Bureau reported in 1998 that the proportion of Americans without health insurance rose to its highest level in a decade: 16.1%. This is 43.2 million fellow citizens, a group in which most of the adults have jobs.

"In a healthy economy, you'd think you would have more people with jobs, and that would tend to increase coverage, so you'd see fewer people uninsured," Census Bureau statistician Robert L. Bennefield said. In the largest states, like Texas and California, the proportion of the uninsured has soared to one in five people.

The HMO industry promised that by moderating premiums, health insurance would be in the reach of more Americans. Yet many employers, particularly small businesses, are now dropping workers and their families from coverage. As noted earlier, premiums are on the rise again. Paul Ellwood predicted in May 1999 that the double-digit increases in premiums will continue "with a vengeance."

The *New York Times* reported in March 1999 that "the uninsured are not the poorest of the poor, who tend to be covered by Medicaid...Of the 43 million Americans without insurance, 75% work at least part time, but are not offered insurance through an employer or cannot afford their contribution. The rest tend to be students, children and early retirees...They are a diverse group, from the chronically ill woman in Harlem who borrows her mother's medicine because she cannot afford her own, to a roofer in Yonkers who is fending off bill collectors, to a young web site designer making about $65,000 a year who takes the calculated risk he will never have to see a doctor at all." A letter to the *New York Times* from Albany Medical Center President James Barba sums up the problem the uninsured pose not only to themselves and their families, but to the nation.

"Having no insurance does not mean that these patients do not get medical attention," wrote Barba. "Regrettably, many wait until they have a health crisis, then present themselves to emergency departments, with the tab picked up by all of us in the form of charity care. This process is highly expensive and inefficient. Prevention and wellness are less expensive. Getting the uninsured assigned to primary-care physicians so that ailments can be treated before they become full-blown crises is a better use of resources, with substantial savings to the country and taxpayers." Mr. Barba's point is not revolutionary. Well-educated policymakers in Washington have recognized this fundamental reality since the turn of the century. The question ever since has been *how* to insure, not *whether* to.

Government-run health insurance programmes like Canada's have been opposed by the American insurance industry. Insurers have effectively used their deep pockets to turn the public against legislative and ballot attempts aimed at preventing private insurers and HMOs from running the system and mandating certain coverage levels. Some segments of the industry, particularly the smaller insurers, spent tens of millions of dollars to defeat President Clinton's proposed national health care system. Opponents of a government dominated system have asked whether Americans wanted the post office as a model for their medicine. Increasingly in the age of HMOs, however, Americans may respond that at least the post office lives up to its commitments and delivers the mail. Of course, it is the Medicare system, not the post office, which is the apt comparison. The Medicare programme operates with a mere 2% for overhead costs. By contrast, private HMOs spend up to 30% for their overhead and profit.

Dr. Carl Weber of White Plains, New York summed up why recent exposés about HMO medicine make a compelling case for the ouster of corporate control of our medical system: "After years of interfering in doctor-patient relations, exacerbating the problem of the uninsured, denying responsibility for medical education and research and rationing health care, health maintenance organisations are refusing to cover the elderly while asking for rate increases. How much more evidence do we need before we realise that managed care is a failed system that should be abandoned?"

Traditionally, there have been two fundamental approaches to "universal health care" — the premise that our society as a whole will insure everyone to protect us all.

First, employers could be required to pay for health care coverage, either through a pay-roll tax or simply by providing coverage for their employees. Such an employer mandate was first proposed by Richard Nixon, so it is hardly a radical idea. The business lobby has fought the employer mandate model on the national level. This model, which currently exists in Hawaii, does not cut private insurers out in favour of a government-run system. In Hawaii, workers and non-workers are covered by the state but given care by private HMOs and health insurers. The state is simply a financing mechanism. Hawaiians, as a whole, seem to feel more satisfied with their HMOs than the rest of Americans, probably because they have the choice of three major competitors and those companies have to compete with quality treatment to win business. President Clinton was working on a similar model for the nation in 1994, but his "managed competition" concept also turned the administration of the system over to HMOs and insurers, which would then tend to compete with each other for healthier customers from the start. Moreover, under "managed competition," too large a percentage of the health care dollar could still go to the companies' profit and overhead rather than to patient care. A second, more straightforward (some might say radical) model is to make the federal government the payer for all health care services, the ultimate administrator and coordinator of a national health care system that is serviced by private health care service givers — doctors, nurses, hospitals, HMOs that "manage care" rather than simply manage money. This system could take many forms. Canada and most European nations have a "single payer" model, which guarantees universal health coverage to all citizens. The problem for many American legislators, whose careers have been sustained by insurance company campaign contributions, is that the insurers are cut out of the deal. The government, not insurers, underwrites risk. More problematic, a single-payer system is typically financed by taxes on employers. Politically, the corporate lobby has teamed with the medical-insurance complex to stop implementation of a single payer health care system. The Republican Congress, of course, needs little encouragement from corporations to oppose any government-run health care plan.

The conservative American Medical Association has opposed such a system in the past because of doctors' fears that a government-run system would cap their fees. But many doctors, having seen the horrors of corporate HMO controls, may yet be ready for a government system that is more reasonable to them. While the public once believed that for-profit companies were more capable of running the health care system, attitudes have changed after prolonged exposure to HMO medicine's vices. A February 1998 poll found that, for the first time, the public believes that not-for-profit companies would do better in running the nation's health care system. In HEDIS patient satisfaction data, not-for-profits also receive much higher ratings. Certainly, there is enough money in the system to insure everyone. A novel proposal by Boston University professor Alan Sager calls for simply freezing all national payments to the health care system from the previous year, and covering every American with a full benefit package from that pool of money.

The trillion dollar health care economy could easily cover every American with comprehensive benefits. Canada, for example, spends 9% of its gross domestic product to insure everyone — while we spend 14% and leave 43 million without insurance. The new American health care system could be coordinated through regional administrations representing all the stakeholders — physicians, patients, payers, and others — that calculate reasonable fees for those providing treatment and monitor utilisation of doctors, as well as watching for fraud. Such a government-run system could be far more efficient than the current one. Sager's system would require no taxes, simply a freeze on payments currently made by employers and other payers. Alternatively the same programme without the co-payments patients now are forced to make would include only a moderate increase in taxes, equal to 5% of health care spending. Such a tax would substitute for the co-pay, which Sager calls, "the tax on being sick." The question Americans and their representatives must ask themselves is which model ensures greater potential for the health of the nation — one run by corporations intent on profits or one run on a non-profit basis and regulated by the government. Ellwood, whose change of heart about his own HMO concept was fostered by his personal experiences with bad medicine, now says, "Uneven health care in the United States is a national disgrace. Ultimately this thing is going to require government intervention. The question is what form government intervention will take. I think whatever it is, it's going to have to be a condition of doing business." Ellwood agrees reform "is not going to come from within" the industry. Two recent independent studies, commissioned by the Massachusetts Medical Society, indicate the waste and overhead in the current system. According to a report in the *Boston Globe*, a Canadian-style single-payer system would save between $170 million and $1 billion annually in the state. Additionally, hundreds of thousands of Massachusetts residents would have coverage; cutting back on the fiscal strain of emergency room medicine. Surely

Massachusetts is not unique in this regard. It is, of course, significant that a state chapter of the AMA would sponsor such a study. The national organisation has been steadfast in its opposition to a single-payer system. American doctors, however, have had both their incomes and freedom to exercise appropriate medicine eroded under for-profit managed care. Any standardized system would reduce the needless paperwork that bogs down medical offices dealing with the vagaries of private insurers. Market enthusiasts should be interested in reducing the inefficiencies in the current system. Certainly American ingenuity can design a public/private partnership to restore the primacy of the doctor/patient relationship and insure more citizens. This will require the elimination of the for-profit insurers from any significant role in American medical care. It will be a bitter political struggle because of the billions of dollars involved. But it may become inevitable as the nation grows older, requires more medical care, and experiences the many flaws of managed care. Never before in American history has there been such an intersection between the interests of the uninsured and of those who pay for insurance but lack peace of mind that they will receive coverage for their medical conditions.

In early 1998, an insured Massachusetts newspaper publisher killed himself, leaving behind a suicide note about his travails trying to get mental health care from his HMO. In the spring of 1998, a distraught man with health insurance parked his truck on a Los Angeles freeway and unfurled a banner that read, "HMOs are in it for the money." Observed by television viewers across the nation, he proceeded to set himself on fire, then discharge a gun in his mouth. Such despair might once have been conceivable among the uninsured, but hardly from the insured in the wealthiest nation in the world. As extreme as the reactions were, too many Americans can identify with the intense frustrations of dealing with HMOs. In June 1999, the *Los Angeles Times* reported that specialists on call with local emergency rooms are now refusing to respond to emergencies for HMO patients because their HMOs do not pay enough. In one case, a surgeon refused to come to the emergency room to operate on a seven month-old who fell and cut her upper lip down to the muscle. A system that manages treatment and costs is needed. But who will run it? The health care crisis that led to the national debate in 1994 over universal health coverage has only been deferred. The rising anger at the deficiencies of HMO medicine is merely a symptom of the same national malaise. Americans will ultimately have to weigh in, once and for all, about the future of their health care system.

If the people do not act, private entrepreneurs certainly will. A high-profile group of investors are already raising venture capital to launch a for-profit HMO patient assistance service and 1-800 hotline, much like the pre-paid road service plan for motorists. For an annual premium or membership fee of about $80 per year, the corporation will provide information about HMOs and limited access to an advocate to help you navigate your HMO when you run into problems — more advanced advocacy packages would cost more. The programme amounts to insurance for your health insurance. Should we need to buy more insurance just to collect on our HMO policy? Can the failure of HMOs to serve us be corrected by more market mechanisms? Will private solutions result in another proliferation of niche businesses that play on patients' fears and are just as exploitive as the HMOs? Unless civil society reasserts itself, the answers may be all too clear.

5

Health Care Reforms: Select Case Studies

GLOBAL DEVELOPMENT CHALLENGES AND HEALTH CARE REFORM

Changes in the role of the state and private sector are seen as central to success of many health care reforms. The article argues for a more focused "stewardship" function of governments in securing equity, efficiency, and quality objectives through more effective policy making (steering), regulating, contracting, and ensuring that adequate financing arrangements are available for the whole population. At the same time, the author argues a strong case for greater private participation in providing health services (rowing). The article reviews related reform trends in health care financing, generation of inputs and service providers. It concludes that reforms often fail, not because of a flawed technical design, but because of other factors. These include a lack of political commitment to change, resistance from vested stakeholders who fear loosing some of their existing benefits, and a failure by policymakers to translate successful aspects of the reforms into something visible that ordinary people and the public can see with their own eyes when next they use the reformed services.

REFORM OF THE HEALTH CARE SERVICE SYSTEM IN ISRAEL 1995-2000

In January, 1995, a national health insurance law was enacted which allowed for the registration of every resident with one of the four public health funds. These funds provide medical services directly to their insured members, or purchase them from public or private hospitals or other health service providers. A basket of medical services was defined which guaranteed readily available comprehensive health care throughout the country. As part of the reform, a number of personal participation charges were established: a nominal fee for medications, and a service charge for a limited number of medical services (visits to specialist doctors, periodic fee for mother and child clinics, participation in the cost of chronic nursing hospitalization). In spite of the Government's commitment to finance the basket of services, the budget is not sufficient to cover costs, and there is an inherent shortfall deliberately introduced into the system by the Ministry of Finance. Since the introduction of the Law the sources for financing the basket of services have been eroded by 16%. Complementary health insurance programmes are being developed by the health funds as well as by private insurance companies. The national expenditure on health is some 8.4% of GDP, with an average annual expenditure of $1,384 per person. 72% of health expenditures are public and 28% private. Life expectancy is continually rising, and stood at 75.9 years for men and 80.1 years for women in 1999. Infant mortality is decreasing: in 1996 the rate was 6.3 per 1,000 live births. There is an ever increasing use of new technologies, even though at the same time there seems to be somewhat of a decrease in customer satisfaction. The achievements of the reform are considerable, but there is need for improvement in the areas of budgeting, return of the employer parallel tax, and in other areas if these achievements are not to be undone. Significant reform in health services in Israel was introduced in January, 1955, following enactment of a compulsory, national health insurance law. The reform guaranteed comprehensive health insurance for all residents of Israel through four already existing health maintenance organizations.

Nature of the Reform

The new national health law obligates every citizen of the State of Israel to register with one of the four public health funds. Each person can choose the fund he/she wishes to join, and if dissatisfied, can also move to another fund once a year. All the health funds are public and are obligated to treat all members registered with them. They are also obligated to provide all health requirements according to a predetermined basket of health services. The health funds provide these services either directly or through purchase from suppliers, such as hospital inpatient treatment. The State is responsible for financing the basket of health services, and allocates the resources to the health funds according to a weighted per capita formula determined by the number of registered members, and by the age of the members. The funds are permitted to offer their members supplementary insurance for services which are not included in the health basket. Israeli citizens are required to pay a health tax based on a rate of between 3.1% - 4.8% of their income.

Scope of Health Services Included in the National Health Insurance Law

The health insurance law ensures equality in comprehensive and readily available health care and medical services, including preventive medicine, a broad immunization programmeme, curative medicine, and diagnostic and medical treatment in community clinics and in inpatient hospital services. Hospitalization includes also maternity care, newborn and premature babies, psychiatry, gerontology, inpatient rehabilitation, and participation in the cost of long term nursing hospitalizaion. Medication is provided at a reduced fee and the directory of medications included in the health basket is updated each year. The Government-set basket of health services encompasses a broad range of medical treatments in the fields of rehabilitation, psychology, physiotherapy, speech therapy, and occupational therapy. It also includes social work services dealing with health problems, occupational health services, preventive dental services for children, diagnosis and treatment of developmental disorders, and medical and psychological treatment for alcohol and drug addiction.

Main Achievements of the Health System

Convenient and accessible community health services have been developed throughout the country. Quality general and specialized hospitals are located in all areas of the country, and health professions have become highly specialized. The life span in Israel has been increasing steadily, and has risen from 70.3 years for men and 73.9 years for women in 1970 to 75.9 years for men and 80.1 years for women in 1999. Infant mortality is in constant decline, and in 1996 it stood at 6.3 per 1000 live births. There has also been increased use of advanced medical technology. New and advanced drugs are constantly being introduced. There is an increase in heart catheterizations for diagnosis and treatment. The proportion of people receiving dialysis is one of the highest in the world. The number of IVF units in the population is also the highest in the world: nearly every general hospital has an IVF unit, and the number of patients is continually increasing. Likewise units for premature babies have been established in all the hospitals, and the number of preemies whose weight is less than 1500g is increasing. There is also an increase in the number of patients who receive artificial respiration in general hospitals, and an increase in intensive care units. Innovative operations are being introduced into the system including kidney, liver and heart transplants, and new treatments for oncology patients. Advanced imaging systems, including MRI, have been introduced in all parts of the country. Clinical and scientific research is very developed and the number of scientific articles published is among the highest in the world. There has been a significant increase in public awareness of advanced health services, and the use of modern communications, including the Internet, have become more and more accepted.

Economic Aspects of the Health System

As a result of the enactment of the new health law, there is ongoing and broad public pressure to add health services, with the result being a continual rise in these services. The national expenditure for health in 1999 stood at 8.4% of the gross national product, with an average expenditure of US $1,384 per person per year. Public expenditure is 72% of the total, while personal expenditure has been rising continually since the law was enacted, and stands at 28% today. Personal expenditure is mainly for supplementary insurance, part - payment for medications, consultation levies for specialists and mother and baby clinics, personal participation for chronic nursing hospitalization and treatment by private doctors. Until 1997 there was a parallel tax wherein employers were obliged to pay 3.8% of the employees salary for health insurance. This tax amounted to about 40–45% of the budget that was needed to administer the health insurance law. In January, 1997, the tax was cancelled by the Treasury and the Government in an effort to encourage production by lowering employer costs. As a result, the portion of the health budget paid by the government has increased and extra payments have been imposed on the public (such as the service charges paid for specialist visits, etc.), and supplementary insurance has increased. In 1999 the Government covered 45% of the total health budget, 26% was covered by the health tax paid by the citizens, and 28% was covered by payment for services (medication, specialist levies etc.)

Role of the Ministry of Health

Generally, there has been no marked change in the role of the health ministry since the enactment of the new health law. The Ministry of Health is concerned with the initiation and updating of health legislation, as well as the planning, licensing, directing and management of the hospitals and health services. It is involved with the management and supervision of the health maintenance organizations, granting licenses for the construction of hospitals, purchasing high-cost medical equipment, ensuring hospitalization services and implementing a comprehensive prevention programmeme. It is also charged with initiating and encouraging programmemes for the advancement of health in Israel, the licensing of medical professionals according to the statutory laws, and the promotion of new technology for the health basket.

Changes in the Level of Public Satisfaction

It has become clear that application of reforms in the health care system is a lengthy and dynamic process, and changes continually need to be made. Unfortunately, information about such changes is not always made known in time to the general public. When public satisfaction level was reviewed, it was evident that the level of satisfaction was high during the first two years of the reform. Since then, however, there has been a definite decline. 13% of the citizens think there should be a total overhaul of the health system, and in general the public perceives the health care system as less efficient than it was before the reform. One of the hypotheses for the decrease in satisfaction is connected to erosion of the budget, the various service payments that are required, and the changes in the level of service.

Main Problems

Ever since the law was first enacted the budget has been insufficient to cover the basket of health services costs. There is an inherent deficit in the health budget which is initiated by the Treasury in order to reduce the increase in the national expenditure for health by reducing costs and improving efficiency. From the enactment of the law in 1995 to 2000 there was a 16% erosion in the Financing of tha basket of services. The health funds are not able to balance their budgets as required by law, and they suffer from operational deficits and difficulties. There are problems maintaining and renewing hospital infrastructures, which often have to rely on donations for implementation. There has also been an increase in personal liability of the public both in direct payments for services included in the basket, such as medication, a service charge for visits to specialists, a service charge for mother and baby clinics, and participation in the cost of chronic nursing hospitalization. This increase in personal liability also increases inequality in providing medical services. It has been shown that 6% of the patients declined treatment because of the payment factor, and 11% did not acquire the prescribed medication. The problem is even more significant among chronic patients who require more services. In addition, supplementary insurance has been initiated to cover those services not provided by the basket of health services. Most supplementary insurance is obtained through the health maintenance organizations, but some private insurance companies also offer supplementary insurance, and today more and more citizens are subscribing in some form.

There are difficulties in updating the basket of health services and in adding new medications. During the first two years of the law, no new medications were added to the basket because of resistance from the Treasury. During the last two years, however, many new and important drugs have been added, although not all that should be. There is a problem with an appropriate budget for the infrastructure of the hospitals, and there has been a decline in creating additional hospital beds. Today the number of beds in general hospitals is 2.27 per 1000 population, 2.7 nursing and rehabilitation beds, and 1.04 psychiatric beds per 1000. The Treasury has endeavored to intervene in the structure of the health system and in setting health policy. It has, as well, sought to enact laws affecting health policy during the passing of the national budget. There is a problem of services for the elderly. Today there are four bodies who are responsible for the elderly: the Ministry of Health, the National Insurance Institution, the Ministry of Labor and Welfare, and the health maintenance organizations. There is a need to provide more resources for the care of the elderly, which would be possible if all the bodies and budgets for their care were merged.. There is also a need to re-institute the parallel tax that will enable an appropriate budget for the health system. The achievements attained by the reforms in the Israeli health system are very significant. Every citizen of Israel is insured for community health services and a high level of hospitalization. With this however, the lack of inherent resources and underbudgeting of the system along with the other problems mentioned, require corrective action in order to prevent a collapse of the health system in the future.

REFORMING HEALTH CARE IN LATIN AMERICA: CHALLENGES AND OPTIONS

The Social Protection Model in Latin America

Because of diverse historical processes, each country in Latin America has developed its own system of social protection. Each is the result of a complex web of economic, political, and cultural forces, and each is unique in the way it turns a set of social values shared by the population into a complex network of institutions responsible for financing, organising, and providing social services delivery, and defining who is entitled to benefits and services. As Flora and Alber (1981) have pointed out in their comparative study of the development of welfare states in Europe and America, modern western systems of social protection originated in the profound economic, political, and cultural changes that accompanied the processes of industrialisation and urbanisation. Alterations in authority patterns, changes in community values, weakening family ties, and the emergence of class identity were some of the features that caused responsibility for the provision of individual and family needs to shift from the private to the public sphere. Thus, the role of the state became more interventionist in order to ensure emerging social rights.

Although the development of social protection has a common origin, the institutional form it takes varies according to prevalent values and previously existing institutions. It is also determined by the dynamics of the power struggle between the important classes and social actors — their goals, strategies, alliances, and ability to organise and create social consensus. Nevertheless, analysts have tried to extrapolate patterns of social protection from specific cases and come up with three ideal types of social protection systems that group similar styles of governmental intervention and organisational arrangement as an outcome of former political choices. These are: the corporatized system, the nationalized system, and the segmented system (Heidenheimer et al. 1983). These indicate, respectively, an insurance-based arrangement, a state-supported system, and a market-based system combined with public assistance.

Some critics feel that such classifications are purely descriptive and cannot properly be called instruments for comparative analysis. Others point out that it is impossible to fit any real system into an ideal type, as an ideal type indicates a prevailing tendency rather than a complex historical dynamic. Although agreeing with this criticism, we cannot deny the utility of identifying the common features in the social-protection development process as a useful tool in the analysis of the present situation of health care systems in Latin America. Other authors recognize the importance of identifying common patterns of social policies, but call attention to the enormous variation in the arrangement of any specific public policy such as health care. This arrangement is the result of political choices on many different issues, such as: ownership of the services; styles of contracting out; means of regulating professional activities; policy-making structure; techniques of intervention; distribution of health care services; and guarantee of access (Heindenheimer et al. 1983, pp. 52-89). That being said, such a classification is undeniably useful in our analysis of the present situation of health care systems in Latin America.

Latin America has traditionally been ruled in a oligarchic way, combining patrimonial mechanisms — the private appropriation of public goods by the elite — with the populist exchange of privileges — the co-opting of workers by government — and the social exclusion of certain groups of people, mainly the poorest.

Nevertheless, social demands have been incorporated by governmental authorities since the beginning of the 20th century, as part of the process of urbanisation and the launch of the industrialisation process. Some of the most powerful, complex, and long-standing social security systems are to be found in the region, especially in those countries considered pioneers: Argentina, Brazil, Chile, and Uruguay (Mesa-Lago 1978). There, social security institutions date back to the turn of the century, and have formed one of the most important channels in the relationship between the populist leader and the urban working class. The government bargained with each labour faction separately, exchanging benefits for political support and thereby deriving its legitimacy. Thus, the social security system was built up on fragmented grounds, with benefits being expanded to the same entitled workers and coverage being enlarged as part of the political game of pressure and bargain, while its financial basis was entirely rooted in taxes and contributions from salaries. The assimilation of the social demands of urban workers has resulted in different levels of social protection in each country, determined mainly by the degree of homogeneity and organisation within the working class (to compare the development of social protection in pioneer countries, see Fleury 1994).

Thus, while social policies and social security systems in Latin America played an important role in the process of state-craft, they did not succeed in spreading civil culture or in extending social coverage. Although the concept of citizenship was based on an egalitarian notion of rights, the concept of social protection in Latin America rested on social and institutional mechanisms of differentiation. Nevertheless, this political give-and-take constituted the first instance in which the demands of the working class were considered in the political arena and incorporated into the government agenda. From this process emerged the main actors in the social policy arena: the technical bureaucracy; middle-class professionals; unionized workers; and, last but not least, the traditional populist politicians. Social protection was rooted in a political system wherein the state played a key role in the industrialisation process by combining industrial protectionism with a controlled political incorporation of urban workers' demands. This apparently strong state interventionism was weakened, however, by the compromises that had to be made with the many conflicting and powerful interests that lent the government legitimacy, but also held it back.

The need to cater to vested interests was responsible, on the one hand, for increased state intervention in social and economic life. On the other hand, it prevented the government from imposing progressive taxes on the productive sector, resulting in chronic fiscal deficit. This populist game, performed by state and society and based on mobilisation and concessions, was paradoxically responsible for both the power and the weakness of the state. As the course of industrialisation proceeded, the ever-growing complexity of the political structure, dissatisfaction due to unfulfilled expectations, and the exacerbation of contradictions between co-optation and control made it impossible to fulfill emerging political and social demands. As a result, the expansion and maturation of the social protection system in the region manifested itself as a crisis that could not be resolved within the existing political framework. With the collapse of populism in the 1960s, social protection institutions suffered an intentional demobilisation of popular participation followed by several attempts to concentrate political power in the hands of a bureaucratic–authoritarian central executive. At that time, the social security institutions controlled by workers in the pioneer countries were about to go bankrupt. The first reform movement carried out by the military dictatorships was to take those institutions out of the hands of the trade unions and put them into the hands of the bureaucracy. This was successfully carried out in Brazil, but failed in Argentina, where the workers were able to keep control of the *obras sociales*, the social security institutions associated with unions.

However, the strengthening of bureaucratic structures was accompanied — to a greater or lesser degree, depending on the country — by a general trend toward de-politicizing social issues, within a context of political suppression and the elimination of representative and organisational channels for expressing social demands. The rupture with the populist style of relationship between state and society did not change the "corporate pact" of power and control over the political actors by the authoritarian governments. However, bureaucracy was substituted for corporate mechanisms of representation and conflict negotiation, which clearly favoured the interests of private entrepreneurs. In the context of social security, this meant private health care providers, whose influence on public policy resulted in a state logic that was predominately private. In any event, each country was left with a stratified health care system whereby workers in the formal market were entitled to social security benefits while the rest of the population received services provided by the ministry of health. This resulted in significant differences in access to and quality of services. Regardless of differences in social protection policies from country to country, it is possible to note some common characteristics. These include:

— duality — some services are provided by the ministry of social security and others by the ministry of health;

— fragmented institutional arrangements that vary in terms of duties and rights according to the bargaining power of the labour group involved;
— centralisation of the social services system, resulting in inefficient service delivery and poor quality services;
— low coverage by a social security system that provides uneven coverage across regions and income classes, and excludes workers in the informal sector; and
— a complex and intricate power structure, dominated by such powerful stakeholders as politicians, bureaucrats, labour leaders, private providers, international suppliers of health-care inputs, and insurance companies.

Despite these common features, health care in Latin America is provided through a wide range of organisational forms of delivery. An attempt to categorize them can be found in the typology adopted by the Inter-American Development Bank (IDB 1996, p. 309).

Segmented Systems are characterized by the coexistence of the following: social security systems covering workers in the formal sector; a health ministry that carries out some public health interventions and provides health care services for the lower and middle classes; and a very large and diverse private sector that covers the richest, the poorest, and, increasingly, the middle class. Mexico was identified as an example of a segmented system.

Contract-Intensive Systems

Contract-Intensive Systems are characterized by the prominence of social security organisations, for which payroll taxes are the major source of financing. These usually involve a formal separation between finance and service provision, and apply a wide range of service-contracting mechanisms. Argentina was identified as an example of this type of system. This typology emphasizes the relationship between payers and providers, but also takes into consideration the ownership of health services. As a descriptive tool, it does not indicate the reasons why a health system assumes this configuration, nor its tendencies to reform it. All of them are identified as facing problems in improving the quality of services and achieving efficiency. Nevertheless, it would be misleading to conclude that the different configurations of the health system in the region are coming to the same point of adopting a standardized reform model.

Subcontracting Systems

Subcontracting Systems are those in which the government plays an important role in mobilizing resources while provision of services is largely private, usually on a fee-for-service basis applied with various degrees of sophistication. Brazil, where abundant private resources complement public efforts, is the only country in the region to approximate such a system.

Integrated Public Systems

Integrated Public Systems are those in which the public system predominates. Financial resources come out of general tax revenues and are allocated to integrated public providers on the basis of installed capacity. Costa Rica was identified as an example of this type of system.

After a Decade of Reforms in Latin America

The structural reforms implemented in the late 1970s and throughout the 1980s saw the emergence of a new style of economic development based on the leading role of private investment and exports, the expansion of private consumption, and a limited role for the state. In most countries of the region, adjusting to the external financial crisis led to regressive income distribution and an acute decline in real wages, further increasing inequality and poverty (O'Donnell and Markovitz 1996). During the 1980s, the "lost decade," the political and social balance achieved during the postwar era of development quickly broke down. Most of the countries emerged from the adjustment period with greater levels of inequality (the exceptions being Colombia, Costa Rica, and Uruguay) and poverty (except for Chile and Uruguay).

Although economic stagnation and inflation were the main factors responsible for poverty and inequality, adjustment measures taken in response to the fiscal crisis also contributed. The new style of development based on increased productivity and competitiveness deepened existing structural problems such as lack of investment capital (national savings), vulnerability to external shocks, and lack of an income distribution policy to cope with poverty and inequality. As the region recovered, experiencing economic growth without inflation, purchasing power increased in some countries and the income distribution structure was altered across the region, with varying effects. Only the high-income groups benefited in Mexico, while all income groups benefited in Chile, Colombia, and Uruguay. In Venezuela, the incomes of all groups deteriorated, while in Argentina and Brazil the middle classes and the poor suffered the greatest losses (Altimir 1994). Only in the mid-1990s would the Brazilian stabilisation policy succeed in reducing inflation and, consequently, poverty.

According to a report by the Inter-American Development Bank (IDB 1997, p. 17), "after falling continually throughout the 1970s, poverty increased dramatically in Latin America during the 1980s. By the end of the decade, the proportion of the population living in moderate poverty had risen to

35%, and the share of the population in extreme poverty had risen to roughly 17%. During the 1990s the poverty rate has declined very slightly, while the number of poor has increased somewhat...." Weak recovery in the 1990s was attributed to the insignificant decline in poverty rates, which may also reflect the manner in which the gains from recovery were distributed (IDB 1977, p. 18). Between 1991 and 1995, per-capita income of the top fifth on the income-earning scale grew by 5%, whereas per-capita income of the middle and lower income groups grew by only 3%. The overall conclusion was that the pattern of income distribution has not shifted in this region, which is noted for having the most unfair income distribution in the world.

Concern about the fragility of the region's economic recovery centered on the fact the that growth that has been restored in some countries is heavily dependent on private foreign investment. Many experts have suggested that privatisation of the social security funds would be the most promising way to raise private savings (Williamson 1997, p. 51) and reduce reliance on public investment.

While other international agencies attribute these failing efforts to reduce poverty to the weakness of the recovery process, a report by the Economic Commission for Latin America and the Caribbean (ECLAC 1996, p. 44) takes a more pessimistic view. The report attributes the persistence of the same pattern of income distribution to some characteristics of the job market, such as the persistently high rate of unemployment, the limited bargaining power of many wage earners, and the increased income gap between workers with different skill levels. Economic recovery is of critical importance to the social sector, because the characteristics of the labour market determine access to social benefits, as well as the possibility of joining a private health insurance plan. The formal job market not only determines salary levels, but also the level of resources collected by social security that are destined for the health sector. Thus, the low income earned by a high proportion of public sector workers — in Bolivia, Honduras, and Venezuela, between 30% and 40% of public sector wage earners were below the poverty line in the mid-1990s (ECLAC 1996) — limits the scope for state reform of social security, and especially affects the social sectors, where the lowest salaries in public administration are to be found. An analysis of the process of change in income distribution and the debate regarding the role played by public policies is revealing. The Chilean case shows that even under sustained economic growth, inequality remains higher now than during the pre-adjustment period, while the examples of Costa Rica and Uruguay show that inequality can decrease as a result of income distribution mechanisms.

The evidence points to the conclusion that there is no economic theory of wealth redistribution, and that the positive results achieved resulted from a set of political policies and increased public expenditure on social services. In other words, Latin America's historic experience illustrates the thesis that, while economic growth is a necessary condition for the struggle against poverty and the reduction of inequities, it cannot by itself improve income distribution. The judicious use of social expenditure is a better way of improving income distribution because it is relative independent from both the level and rate of economic expansion. The last period of crisis and the implementation of structural economic adjustment measures led to reduced employment and wage levels and increased poverty and inequality throughout the region. Nevertheless, it did not reverse the long-range trend toward improved social conditions. Rather, it reduced the rate of social improvement, particularly in the areas of educational coverage, water and sanitation services, child mortality, and life expectancy at birth. Continued improvement in social conditions must be attributed to the social service networks established in several countries during the period of economic expansion and to socio-demographic characteristics associated with the accelerated rate of urbanisation.

Fertility rates have declined rapidly in Latin America since the mid-1970s, reducing population growth and eliminating the threat of overpopulation. The challenge is now to take advantage of this opportunity by improving the quality and coverage of social programmemes, particularly with respect to young people living in poverty. In addition to reduced fertility rates, the region has experienced significant economic and social changes in the recent decades, mainly, an intense process of urbanisation and the aging of the population. Both phenomena have altered the demand for health care, since urban demands are more visible than the rural demands, and the aging of the population has redrawn the epidemiological profile. To the typical diseases of underdevelopment have been added those prevalent in industrialized societies: cardiovascular disease, chronic illness, accidents, and violence.

In Latin America, the health sector is a powerful economic force, employing about 5% of the economically active population (EAP). Expenditure on health represents on average 5.7% of gross national product (GNP) in the countries of the region (CEPAL 1994). However, public expenditure on health care accounts for only 49% of total health expenditure in the region; private expenditure for 50% and foreign development assistance for the remaining 1% (Govindaraj et al. 1995). In terms of public expenditure on health care, the region does not compare favourably with the world average. Public expenditures on health care in the region is US $121 per person per year, or 2.2% of GNP, less than half of the world average of about US $323 per person per year (World Bank 1993). While the level of public spending on the social sector increased during the early 1990s in most countries in the region (ECLAC 1996, p. 79), the increases varied greatly between countries. In some countries, expenditures now exceed the levels prevailing in the 1980s. This is the case in Argentina, Chile, Colombia, Costa Rica, Mexico, Panama, Paraguay, and Uruguay. In other countries, expenditures show an upward trend, but have not yet regained early 1980s' levels. Such is the case in Bolivia, Ecuador, and El Salvador. Social expenditures in yet other countries, such as Brazil, Guatemala, Honduras, and Nicaragua, have fluctuated or declined slightly. Moreover, most increased public spending in the region occurred in the areas of education and social security, rather than health.

During the 1980s, reduced public spending was accompanied by an increase in health expenditures on the part of families, enterprises, and nongovernmental organisations (NGOs). The NGO contribution to the region's health financing was significant, totaling US $6 billion between 1980 and 1989. In poorer countries, this contribution was similar to or even exceeded that of national governments. As a result of reduced public spending, public health services tended to deteriorate, the technological gap between public and private hospital services widened, and the efficiency and effectiveness of publicly managed and provided health care declined. This was accompanied by a growth in services supplied by the private insurance sector, which increased significantly both in affiliation and number of hospital beds. Thus the pattern of supply and consumption moved toward greater involvement of the private sector in health care delivery. In addition to changing market dynamics, there also occurred in Latin America a great transformation in the social fabric and institutional political framework. Since the 1970s, the old relationship between state and society that had developed during the early years of industrialisation — known as the "corporate pact" — showed itself incapable of encompassing the complex and pluralistic network of political actors that emerged as part of the urbanisation and industrialisation processes. Grassroots social movements and NGOs flourished in the region, becoming a channel for organising and representing interests that did not fit into the old political order. Even traditional political actors, such as trade unions and entrepreneurs, developed new forms of organisation and representation, clearly demonstrating the insufficiency not only the old structure but also the political party and electoral systems. Moreover, the increase in unemployment and changes in the work process have weakened the power of the trade unions in the region and limited their ability to control or implement social policies.

The transition to democracy in many countries of the region in the late 1980s changed the existing pattern of authority into a scene of conflict, where consensus, as well as the institutional framework of democracy, had yet to be built up. In this new context, social and grassroots demands had to be considered in the political arena, some of them becoming part of the government agenda. At the same time, however, economic adjustment measures imposed tremendous cuts in public spending, emphasizing the contradictions between necessities and constraints. Deepening inequity, the "urbanisation of poverty," and the failure of the state to guarantee even minimal economic and social functions (a stable currency, taxation, education, health, and housing), led to unprecedented urban social breakdown, manifesting itself in violence, criminality, lawlessness, and the proliferation of drug trafficking such as can be read about any day in the regional press. The emerging individualist, or self-centered, system of values acts as a barrier to keeping or developing solidarity, destroying the political and family ties that traditionally provided the poor with social and economic support. Another aspect of individualism, that of consumers' free choice, has had the effect of reducing the power of the bureaucracy to determine the nature of public goods to be offered and the manner of their consumption.

Some Issues in Comparative Analysis

Over the last decade, health care systems in several Latin American countries have undergone a number of organisational changes in line with the worldwide trend toward health sector reform. Such changes were perceived as an answer to the financial crisis of the 1980s, an attempt to make health care institutions more effective and as a way of adapting to the more sweeping process of economic restructuring and the rethinking of the role of the state. The first question one has to ask about these processes of health care reorganisation is whether or not they can rightly be considered as sanitary reform (health reform). Of course the answer will depend on what is meant by the latter. Sanitary reform encompasses changes at both the institutional and the policy levels, transforming both prevailing values and the authority system that is designed to govern individual actions. These transformations are processed in a sustainable way, no matter whether the strategy has been piecemeal or comprehensive. Reforms are supposed to affect crucial features of health care organisation, altering access and utilisation, as well as institutional arrangements and political and economic power-sharing among the various actors in the field.

The political process of sanitary reform in Italy and Brazil has inspired a definition that emphasizes the political and the institutional changes (Fleury 1989). Sanitary reform refers to the process of transforming the laws and the institutional arrangements responsible for protecting the health of citizens, and corresponds to an effective displacement of political power toward less-advantaged groups. The concrete expression of this change is reflected in the establishment of a universal right to health care and the creation of a national health system headed by the state. The same emphasis on the political aspect is evident in another concept of sanitary reform (Berlinguer et al. 1988, p. 131), although it also calls attention to the transformations of the health care model and services. When we aim to broaden the equality of citizens with respect to health care; to displace the power of the few to the many; to change productive technology and individual behaviour in a healthy way; to recycle the services, the technical interventions, the treatment and prevention of disease; and to drive conscientiously other transformation processes (without which any reform would stay isolated and be defeated), we will clearly face many difficulties and huge resistance. Consensus is the most important weapon to overcome them. In other words, after the profound changes in the health sector in Europe in the first half of the century, the discussion about sanitary reform acquired a political meaning in terms of:

— rebuilding the power structure by promoting sanitary conscience (health awareness) and organising a new hegemony;

— altering the legal and institutional health care apparatus, with the state guarantee of universal right and access to a national health system; and

— shifting from a curative to a more preventive orientation, accompanied by more adequate treatment.

The missing point in this case relates to the microeconomic aspects of health care system organisation, i.e. the financing and organising health care units. Recently, this matter has become paramount for reformers, changing the concept of sanitary reform into that of health care reform. This new wave of health sector reform started in a different context, in the middle of the economic crisis of the 1970s. It was prompted by the increasing cost of health care services and the more complex and expensive demands made on the health system by an aging population. In response to national fiscal crises and to the difficulty of financing health care services, health sector reform is underway or under consideration in countries throughout the world. Although it is difficult to define precisely, Berman (1995, p. 15) acknowledges that the term "health sector reform" has wide appeal. He defines it as "sustained, purposeful change to improve the efficiency, equity, and effectiveness of the health sector." He refers to the health sector as all the policies, programmemes, institutions, and actors that together make up the organised effort to treat and prevent disease. In a comparative analysis of seven countries that are members of the Organisation for Economic Co-operation and Development (OECD), Hurst (1991, p. 14) tries to find similarities in terms of some set of objectives as expressed in their health policies. They areas follows:

— individuals should have adequate and equal access to health care;

— payment should be linked to an individual's ability to pay;

— health expenditure should consume an appropriate fraction of GDP (macroeconomic efficiency);

— the mix of services provided should maximise health outcome and consumer satisfaction for the share of GDP expended (microeconomic efficiency);

— consumers should be free to choose arrangements from both the public sector and the private sector; and

— doctors and other providers should be given the maximum freedom compatible with the attainment of these objectives.

The concept of reform that grew out of the attempt to overcome the crisis in the welfare state focused on the need to increase the efficiency and reduce the cost of health services. It also proposed changes in the role of the state and private providers, as well as a shift in the status of the user. This concept of reform sees the state as having a minimum responsibility while assuring the providers their autonomy and dealing with the users as consumers with freedom of choice. Equity of access and protecting patients against financially debilitating payments for health care are also on the agenda, mostly in the developed countries although not in the United States. The discourse of empowerment that accompanied the first reform movement has been replaced by one that emphasizes rationality and competition. According to Chernichovsky (1995), the systematic functions involved in the new generation of reforms are the financing of care, the organisation and management of the consumption of publicly funded care, and the provision of care. Reforms in line with this paradigm attempt to combine the advantages of universality, efficiency and consumer satisfaction by offering universal access to a basic package of care through decentralized, mainly private, systems of delivery. To achieve this goal, the two functions of financing and provision must be separated because the first is guided by a public principle whereas the second is based on competition. International agencies and experts from the region took part in a special meeting in 1995, In order to build a regional agenda for health sector reform in

Latin America (Health Sector Reform Seminar 1995). Participants in the seminar defined health sector reform as, "a process aimed at introducing substantive changes into the relationships between and roles performed by the different agencies involved in the health sector, with a view to increasing equity of benefits, efficiency in management, and effectiveness in satisfying the health needs of the population." The objectives of health sector reform for the region were identified as follows:

- to improve the health and living conditions of all the inhabitants of the Americas;
- to become, along with justice, well being, and equity, one of the pillars of development in the region;
- to reduce health status inequalities, improve access to good quality health services, and foster shared responsibility between institutions, individuals, and communities;
- to modernize and decentralize the organisation and operation of public institutions providing health services;
- to balance the public and private health sectors in order to achieve a synergy in their efforts; and
- To ensure that sufficient financial resources are available to the sector at a sustainable level to accomplish the aforementioned objectives.

The emphasis is on regional problems and strategies, such as promoting equality of access; improving the quality of health services; modernizing the state and decentralizing the provision of services; and gathering resources to operate and finance the health care system. Nonetheless, the concept of health sector reform proposed for Latin America neglects some important aspects of the health sector, such as the development of science and technology, human resources training, and the ever-increasing proliferation of curative treatments. In this research project, we have avoided choosing an existing concept of health sector reform, because we felt that it would lead to an analytical bias in favour of one concept or another. We have also tried to avoid considering health sector reform as a simple rearrangement of organisational variables such as financing, provision, and coverage. Rather, we have chosen to conceptualize health sector reform in terms of the following dichotomies:

— universal versus segmented policies;
— mechanisms of solidarity versus equity between contributions and benefits;
— integrated systems versus fragmented systems; and
— decision-making processes based on participation versus decision-making processes based on competition.

Actual health sector reforms can be expected to fall somewhere along the continuum between the two extremes, permitting many different arrangements. Also, a tendency in one direction or another will be restrained by the existing institutional and political organisation, tending to add to the diversity and complexity of the reforms. We agree with the conclusion of the Health Sector Reform Seminar (1995, p. 11) about the diversity of processes in the region. The objectives, scope, and substance of reform, as well as the strategies and mechanisms adopted for their implementation, vary markedly. Some reforms are comprehensive, simultaneously encompassing the organisation, the financing and the resources of the sector as a whole. Other reforms are intended to implement only partial changes among some of the institutions or roles of the health sector. In some cases, reform involves the promotion of greater private sector participation in health, whereas, in others making decentralized and democratic government more responsible is what has been attempted. One way to avoid the problem of diversity when comparing the reforms is to analyse the purposeful change made by governmental authorities, and expressed in legal instruments. But this may be misleading. Kroneman and Zee (1997) call attention to the troublesome task of investigating health policy reforms at the national level, because of the difficulty of establishing when a certain policy change took effect and of determining the content of the reform. The difficulties are due to regional variations in a decentralized system, as well as to the fact that reforms are a gradual rather than a straightforward process. Moreover, deliberate vagueness in national policies is used by reformers as a means of avoiding confrontation with health care providers and other actors, and of creating broad support for the reform.

Nevertheless, a framework can be constructed that avoids these pitfalls by focusing on the accomplishments and problems associated with various national experiences currently underway. For example, in examining the purpose, content and scope of the sanitary reform processes in Argentina, Brazil, and Mexico, it is possible to discern a common trend toward modifying the relationships between public and private agents and between different levels of government. In our comparative framework, we decided to concentrate on the changing aspects of the health care system, thereby focusing on the main point of consensus in different concepts and processes of sanitary reform. Both those processes that emphasize the political aspect of reform and those that emphasize its managerial content have in common the fact that all the intended changes should appear in the organisational structure of the health care system. Although the decision to concentrate the comparative study on the health care system may avoid problems related to the definition of reform, other comparative issues persist because health systems comprise many complex interactions permitting innumerable variations in policy and in delivery and control mechanisms. This complexity leads many authors to doubt the possibility of accomplishing comparative analysis at all.

Nevertheless, many studies have attempted to compare national health care systems, mostly using a health service model. The health service model develops criteria to group national health systems on the basis of a cross-sectional assessment of each of their components. (Ellencweig 1992, p. 25). One weakness of this model is its implicit effort to reduce the explanation of a multifaceted health care system to one or two variables. Its other weakness is that it disregards trends over time. Roemer (1977) is the most outstanding advocate of the health services approach. He distinguishes the evolution of health systems by identifying four major attributes: historical perspective, political process, socioeconomic environment, and cultural characteristics. His comparative study (cited by Light 1997, p. 109) presents a dynamic model of common elements based on five factors: resources, economic support, organisation, management, and delivery of services. Traditional taxonomy of national health systems was based on ownership, including accountability for financing and provision. This classification could accommodate many different variables, from societal values to market or institutional arrangements involved in a national mandatory insurance scheme. More recently, with the increased complexity of health systems, many different relationships have developed between the government, mandatory and voluntary insurance schemes, and private providers. Thus classification of health systems by ownership is no longer considered useful. Instead, more recent typology is based on the functions performed by each component of the system: financing, regulation, organisation, and provision (Lodoño and Frenk, 1997). The health care system is analysed in terms of its capacity to integrate either populations or institutions. With respect to populations, integration means the extent to which different groups are allowed access to every institution in the health system. Regarding institutions, integration refers to the arrangements for carrying out the functions. Upon this framework, Lodoño and Frenk (1995) created the following typology of health systems models in Latin America:

— the unified public model, featuring vertical integration of institutional functions and horizontal integration of populations;
— the segmented model, featuring vertical integration of institutional functions and segregation of populations;
— the fragmented model, featuring separation of institutional functions and horizontal integration of populations; and
— the atomized private model, featuring separation of institutional functions and segregation of populations.

This new way of classifying the components by function is based on two premises: the necessity of separating the financing and provision functions, and the existence of more than one type of public-private mix. The typology is used as a way to reach a proposal for a new arrangement for health care systems in Latin America called "structured pluralism."

Gonzalez-Block (1997, p. 201) identifies this approach to comparative analysis as the use of an "ideal type" model, abstracted from the institutional arrangements and processes found in existing health care systems in industrialized countries so as to maximise certain desirable attributes. He also points out some problems in the use of an ideal type, for example, the possibility of oversimplifying existing institutions and actors, as well as the normative aspects implicit in it. "Structured pluralism" is put forward as the best arrangement to achieve efficiency, responsiveness, accountability, and solidarity through an appropriate mix of public and private financing, delivery, and regulation. However, this arrangement tends to conceal the political and ideological aspects by treating any possible arrangement of relations and variables as a matter of technical expertise. In addition to the health services approach, Ellencweig (1992, p. 22) identified two other kinds of taxonomy used in the comparative analysis of health systems: the health policy approach and the epidemiological model. The politico-economic approach is a policy-oriented model that has been adjusted to distinguish between national health systems based on the assumption that they really do manifest clear-cut ideologies (Ellencweig 1992, p. 29). As distinct from the static health services approach, the politico-economic approach encompasses historical, political and economic processes, although it fails to provide concrete tools for comparing the elements of health care systems.

The epidemiological approach applied to comparative health system analysis works with multiple dimensions, such as the social (covering political, socio-cultural, economic, and demographic elements), the institutional, and the individual. This multilevel analysis assigns causal effects to a variety of factors and is used to study the interrelationships between several effects and their causes (Ellencweig 1992, p. 35). Despite the importance of multilevel analysis and the historical perspective, it would be difficult to establish direct causal links between different political and economic orientations and the institutional arrangements of health care systems. The same holds true for linkages between the institutional and the individual levels. To cope with the difficulties involved in implementing a cross-national multidimensional comparative analysis, Ellencweig (1992, p. 36) proposed the construction of a modular approach. The modular model is made up of a number of separate modules which can be grouped together as needed.... Comprehensive cross?comparisons of systems might be desirable but are often beyond reach. The study of longitudinal trends is similarly limited. However, we can still make several comparisons that can be valuable on a narrower perspective, even when only a few modules are available for comparison. The big advantage of the modular approach is that it can be used for solving problems of various sizes. From the many modules making up the system, appropriate modules may be chosen for each problem to be solved. The weakness of this approach is due to the inherent difficulty of linking the results found in several modules. Even so, the approach seems useful in comparative analysis, in that it permits different levels of comparison, from the suggestion of analogical association to the establishment of causal links based on evidence.

Methodological Options

For the reasons described earlier, we have adopted a modular approach to study the ongoing health care reform processes in Argentina, Brazil, and Mexico in a comparative manner. The consist of a politico-economic analysis of the macroeconomic and social transformations in the region over the last 20 years and describe the way that these may have affected the institutional arrangement of the health care system. The theoretical model underlying the design of the study assumes that each society, at different times in its development, assigns priority to certain organisational forms and regulatory mechanisms of the health care system, associating these instruments with values such as equity, freedom of choice, and efficiency. The intention is not to establish causal links between macro socioeconomic process and health care system reform. The presumption is rather that health care systems are driven by values, institutional dynamics, political choices, technical interventions, popular demand, and pressure from actors with different degrees of control over important resources in the health care arena. The political, institutional, and health environment into which health care reforms were introduced in each of the three countries, using a politico-economic approach. To maintain a historical perspective, we reconstructed the background influences and primary factors that could have affected the launch and political meaning of health care reform processes. The legislative and administrative tools used to effect health care reform, as well as the strategy adopted to implement it. The implementation process itself is the result of powerful dynamics among different actors in the health care arena, representing several vested interests. Usually, the result is a complex process of give and take, sometimes yielding results that differ profoundly from what was originally intended. The evaluation of the overall process is intended to point out the stresses and contradictions, as well as the differences between rhetoric and reality, in each country. The discussion of dissimilar realities is limited to a careful description of the reform processes founded on a common analytical framework, although the method could allow the identification of similarities and differences in terms of general trends. To overcome the criticism related to the use of a highly conceptual model and the lack of tools for comparing elements making up the health system, we decided to complement these studies with a second comparative module.

A health care systems approach and apply it in each country. To avoid the tendency to adopt a simplistic model based on a one-dimensional typology, we decided to build a comparative framework of health systems, encompassing the main dimensions that are likely to be affected by existing reform processes. In each dimension, we grouped important variables, aiming to characterize the methods of financing, regulation, organisation, and provision. The model adopted in this component of the study includes the reconstruction of such interactions in a historical perspective, focusing on changes in the following:

- the regulatory capacity of the main actors within the health sector;
- prevalent organisational forms characterizing services with regard to ownership, professional profile, and resource allocation;
- sources of financing, risk-sharing options, financing methods, and monetary flows; and
- conditions of provision of services to different population groups, and the results in terms of equity, accessibility, and efficiency.

The static characteristic of the health system approach could be minimized by illustrating the health care system at different points in its development along the reform process. Using the same framework (financing, regulation, organisation, and provision), we describe the health care system arrangements in the 1970s and the 1990s, to achieve a comparative picture of each system's organisational and institutional transformation. To understand the dynamics of the reform process through the relationships and interactions between the main actors, we adopted the model proposed for OECD study of comparative sanitary reforms

(Hurst 1991). It identifies five principal actors in health care systems:

— consumers-patients;
— first-level providers;
— second-level providers;
— insurers or third-parties; and
— government as regulator of the system.

One can analyse the transformations that have occurred in recent years in the health sector through the changes in the relations between the main actors, as described. Using the interactive approach, we will analyse the links between: financiers and providers of health care; the population and financing entities; and patients and providers. Finally, we will refer to the instances and regulating methods operating in the systems analysed. In a comparative analysis of several countries implemented by the Organisation for Economic Co-operation and Development, seven basic arrangements were identified (OECD 1992, p. 19-27), according to the flow of patients, the flow of money, and the relationships of authority:

— the voluntary, out-of-pocket model where there is no insurance and health care is based on direct, out-of-pocket, fee-for-service transactions between consumers and primary- or secondary-level providers;
— the voluntary reimbursement model based on the full or partial reimbursement of patients for medical care bills within a private voluntary insurance scheme;
— the public reimbursement model based on the same reimbursement principles as the above, but within a public compulsory insurance scheme;

- — the voluntary contract model whereby independent providers supply services to the insured under private contractual agreements, mostly free of charge;
- — the public contract model based on a compulsory public insurance where independent providers supply services to the insured under capitation or fee-for-service payments;
- — the public integrated model based on a public compulsory insurance as above, but delivered by non-independent providers, usually paid through salaries and prospective budgets; and
- — the voluntary integrated model based on private voluntary insurance, delivered by salaried providers with prospective budgets.

This characterisation of models of interaction not only allows us to compare the basic design of various systems, but also the dynamics of their transformation with regard to some of the most important dimensions of health policy. It can be expected that whenever the health care system is segmented rather than integrated, as in Latin America, parallel policies, institutions, and systems for different population groups will result. The possibilities for comparison between the three countries are restricted at the outset by the unique configuration of the health care system in each country. Nevertheless, similar trends may be evident even if they occur in different organisational settings. Our hypothesis is that the reshaping of health care systems over the last 20 years has broadening freedom of choice between providers, rendered coordination more difficult, and aggravated existing inequities with respect to the accessibility, utilisation, and quality of services in the health care system. Another important criticism of the use of the health care system approach is that its national focus limits

its ability to discern variations imposed by ongoing tendencies toward decentralisation and privatisation. The third module is a quantitative study of the utilisation of health care systems in three cities: Rosario, Argentina; Rio de Janeiro, Brazil; and Mexico City, Mexico. Questions may be raised regarding the ability to draw conclusions about the national health system based on a study of one city. Aside from practical considerations, our justification for adopting this approach is that the selected cities exhibit the main features of the national health care systems of which they are a part.

Service use, measured at the individual level, was the key outcome. The quantitative approach used in this module allowed us to look for causal links between the configuration of the health care system and the utilisation of services. However, being cross-sectional in nature, such an approach does not lend itself to attributing causal relationships between variations in service use and reform measures. For this study, we used a theoretical model akin to Andersen and Newman's behavioural model on health care utilisation (Andersen and Newman 1973) and applied it to service use specific to four tracer conditions. A survey was designed to reveal the causal relations between three sets of components of the Andersen and Newman model:

- The predisposing component comprises those factors that existed before the onset of illness: a set of demographic, socio-cultural, cognitive, and attitudinal variables that are postulated as personal factors that identify the potential risk group but cannot be modified through health policies.
- The enabling component consists of the organisational and financial factors that affect the individual's ability to access a given service.

- The need component expresses the individual's perceived need for care.
- The predicted relations between these components are as follows:
- Predisposing variables may influence health services utilisation through their effect on the enabling component and on the need variable, as well as directly.
- Enabling variables influence utilisation directly and also through the need variable.
- The need variable influences utilisation directly.

Path analysis allows us to divide the correlation observed between variables into direct and indirect effects. The hypothesis for our quantitative study is that the health care system will be more or less equitable depending on the weight of the enabling component in the utilisation of health care services by patients. The higher the weight of the enabling component, the less the utilisation of services is based on perceived need or predisposing factors, and hence the more inequitable the system. The tracer conditions were selected taking into account the epidemiological characteristics of the population under study; the biological characteristics of the tracer condition, determining the form and frequency of utilisation of health care resources; the type of attention required; and the discretionary or non-discretionary use of services. The selected tracers were diarrhea, hypertension, pregnancy, and delivery.

THE CONTEXT AND PROCESS OF HEALTH CARE REFORM IN ARGENTINA

This study will present a historical perspective on the reform of health services in Argentina. First, it will analyse the macro socioeconomic and political context within which the reform took place. Next, it will trace the legislative and institutional development of the reform. Finally, it will present a political analysis of the particular conditions in the health sector that limit the ability of the state to regulate it. The reform of the health services system (HSS) in Argentina came about as a consequence of the grave economic crisis of the 1980s. At that time, the role of the state in the economy and social welfare was shaped by the need to cope with the explosive growth in demand that arose from the recovery of democratic institutions. As well, over the past 15 years, Argentine society had undergone profound changes to its economic structure and political system, which generated particular problems with respect to social integration.

The impact of the crisis on Argentine society was similar to that which occurred elsewhere in Latin America, being characterized by a marked drop in production levels, accelerated inflation, a drastic reduction in economic activity, and high unemployment. External indebtedness imposed the need to generate ever larger trade surpluses, while maintaining a balanced budget to ensure monetary stability. Other effects of the crisis included increasing instances of social exclusion, the pauperisation of the middle classes, and an alarming spread of extreme poverty. The most apt word to describe Argentine policies in the 1980s is "adjustment": adjustment of the productive apparatus to world market conditions; adjustment of the financial system to production levels; and adjustment of state spending to available resources. The unavoidable modernisation of the state reinforced the socially exclusive features of the economic policies adopted by emphasizing cutbacks in personnel and spending without directing available resources toward social programmemes. Beginning in 1991, the success of the Convertibility Planhttp://archive.idrc.ca/books/focus/923/

s2c02.htm - _ftn1 stimulated the recovery of internal and external investment, making greater flexibility in spending possible. Important changes had taken place in the structure of the productive apparatus, as well as in social and institutional forms of organisation.

The most salient features of the new economy were as follows: the consolidation of new economic and financial groups representing local capital; the development of specialized natural resource-intensive industries; and the redefinition of the terms of entry into international trade, particularly in matters concerning the profile of exports. In addition there have been important changes in the world market, in trade union activity, and in the production of certain public services, as a result of new strategies of deregulation, privatisation, and the opening up of the economy. No less important were the changes in the political system, which have not been confined to the recovery of democracy. President Menem's administration has continued the "presidential" tradition whereby the executive takes the leading role and parliament shows little initiative. The Menem administration benefited from much better conditions for untroubled government than its predecessors and was able to take advantage of a favourable international climate and obtain support for its transformation policies from large national and international investors. Other factors that worked in the government's favour and helped get the reforms underway were as follows: the support of the supreme court of justice, which enabled the President to legislate by means of Decretos de Necesidad y Urgencia (emergency decree); the inability of the opposition to appear as a feasible alternative; the weakening of the trade unions; and, in particular, the fragmentation of the labour movement.

These policies had a number of positive results in terms of macroeconomic indicators: inflation control; high investment rates; a large growth in the gross domestic product (GDP) between 1991 and 1994; an increase in productivity in specific sectors; a significant increase in the export of goods and services; and recovered equilibrium in terms of balance of trade and balance of payments. Negative aspects included a contraction of the labour market, with accompanying unemployment and underemployment; difficulties in achieving fiscal balances in 1995, 1996, and 1997; and excessive dependence on international financial flows due to an underdeveloped local capital market and insufficient domestic savings. In the area of social policies in general, and those relating to the health sector in particular, there were important differences between the policies pursued by the Alfonsin administration (1983–89) and that of President Menem (1989 to the present). In the former case, rationalisation and cost-cutting strategies were oriented according to guidelines advocating strong state intervention, maintaining the bases of solidarity, a tendency toward universality, and the participation of business, trade unions, and professional associations. By contrast, the present administration has emphasized deregulation, privatisation, and contracting freedom in matters related to the organisation and financing of health care, especially since implementation of the 1991 Convertibility Plan. At the same time, It has put into effect plans to focus on and support social demands in specific areas on the basis of agreements reached with the World Bank.

Background Influences

In Argentina, the health services system (HSS) was historically made up of three relatively independent subsystems: public, private, and social security. From the 1960s onward, each of these subsystem and the relationships between them underwent considerable changes, resulting in the HSS that is now the subject of reform. The HSS that existed between the 1960s and the 1990s was characterized first and foremost by the decline of the public subsystem — the one responsible for providing health care to the poor — both in terms of financial and material resources and in technical and managerial efficiency. This decline was compensated for by the growth of the social security sector and by an expansion of services on the part of the private sector.

The social security sector was composed until recently of a large number (about 370) of institutions called *obras sociales* that acted as health insurance funds for workers and their dependents. The *obras sociales* originated and grew under the trade unions' control. The system was institutionalized in 1970 with the passing of Law 18.610. This law made it mandatory for employers and employees to contribute to the *obra social* administered by their trade union. The *obras sociales* provided health care to their beneficiaries in two ways: through their own health services and by contracting facilities from the private sector. This form of organisation became the basis of the HSS, which gradually grew more varied and fragmented as each trade union developed its own health care service, or subcontracted it from the private sector, with little regulation or coordination by the state. In less than a decade, a considerable expansion of private facilities occurred, measured in terms of physicians, hospitals, and technology. In the absence of state regulation, the HSS fell under the control of two large groups of associations: the *obras sociales*, on the demand side, politically represented by the Confederación General del Trabajo (CGT, general labour confederation); and the medical federations and private hospital owners' organisations, on the supply side. Since the 1960s, private health care institutions have been grouped into large federations at the national level comprising physicians, biochemists, pharmacists, dentists, and providers of services for inpatient care. Until very recently, these large tertiary federations, representing provincial federations and local associations, have maintained control of the power to contract with the *obras sociales*.

The Instituto Nacional de *Obras sociales* (INOS, national institute of *Obras sociales*,) was the state agency responsible for managing the system. Its main function, according to Law 18.610, was to regulate the operation of the *obras sociales*, so as to reduce the large differences in financial capacity between them and to guarantee their beneficiaries access to a basic set of health services. The INOS was responsible for monitoring contracts between financing institutions and the large physicians' federations. The regulatory capacity of the INOS proved insufficient to reduce the inequalities between *obras sociales*, however, and they continued to vary in terms of number of beneficiaries, institutional regime, consumption profile, cost structure, and service model. The result was a mosaic of arrangements, differing from region to region and union to union. No sooner was the system introduced in 1970, than attempts were made to reorganise it. The proposed reforms attempted, on the one hand, to assure better use of resources and a more equitable distribution of benefits. On the other hand, they sought to take control of the *obras sociales* away from the trade unions, which had gradually become a source of political and economic power, in many cases, to the detriment of their specific function. Attempts to reorganise the system in 1973, 1978, and 1985 failed due to concerted opposition on the part of the CGT. With the passing of Laws 23.660 and 23.661 in 1989, modifications were made in the norms regulating the system, but no changes were made to the fundamental parameters governing its organisation. By this time, financial deficits were seriously hampering the operation of the *obras sociales*, prompting them to raise their members' contributions on several occasions. Law 23.661, the purpose of which was to lay the legislative basis for the development of a national health insurance scheme, put the system under control of a new agency dependent on the Ministerio de Salud y Acción Social de la Nación (MSAS, ministry of health and social action). The Administración Nacional del Seguro de Salud (ANSSAL, national health insurance administration), as it was called, proved as incapable of imposing order as its predecessor, INOS. The new law also modified the system's nomenclature, now referring to the heterogeneous group of *obras sociales* as "health insurance agents." This initiative was based on the expectation that under the control of ANSSAL, the system would gradually expand through the voluntary incorporation of independent provincial *obras sociales*, as well as some mutual aid societies.

To complete this summary of the situation of the HSS at the time the reform began, it is necessary to take a look at private health insurance institutions, called Empresas de Medicina Pre-paga. These institutions originated in the late 1960s, but were of limited significance up until the beginning of the 1980s. From then on they grew in importance and became a supplement to, or a substitute for, the *obras sociales* as far as the higher-income segments of the population were concerned. The private health insurance institutions were as heterogeneous as the *obras sociales*. Some were organised by physicians' associations and large private hospitals with a view to increasing the number of options for financing their services. Others were companies that functioned exclusively as financing agencies, subcontracting private services for their clients' coverage. To complicate matters, some of these companies acquired facilities of their own, with a view to becoming more competitive.

The Reform Process: Formulation of Reform Policy

The hyperinflationary period of 1989–90 paved the way for reforms that went well beyond the framework of the health services system (HSS). The main instruments for transforming the Argentine socioeconomic system were the State Reform Law and the Economic Emergency Law, passed in 1989 as part of the agreement that resulted in Raul Alfonsín handing over power to Carlos Menem before the scheduled date. The State Reform Law declared practically all state enterprises to be subject to privatisation and modified the regime governing public services. The Economic Emergency Law firmly tackled the issue of reducing public spending. It suspended all subsidies and grants affecting the national treasury, promotion regimes for mining and industry, and all regulations restricting foreign investment. At the same time, it authorized the executive to divert to other uses funds having a specific purpose; to revise contracts with public employees, to modify the labour indemnity system; and to set up a penal regime for noncompliance with tax obligations. The reform strategies adopted a course decidedly favouring deregulation of the economy.

With respect to health, in 1991, the Ministerio de Economía de la Nación (ministry of the economy) launched a strategy aimed at centralizing social security contributions, with a view to facilitating control of these resources by state officials. To this end, the government established the Sistema Unico de Seguridad Social (SUSS, unified social security system), under Article 85 of the Economic Deregulation Decree (2.284/91). SUSS was dependent upon the Ministerio de Trabajo y Seguridad Social de la Nación (MTSS, ministry of labour and social security), and established the Contribución Unica de Seguridad Social (CUSS, unified social security contribution) to combine social security and health care contributions. The law gave SUSS the power to collect, administer, and supervise the distribution of all payroll deductions through the Fondo Solidario de Redistribución (FSR, solidarity redistribution fund), created under Decree 2.741/91. The percentage of funds destined for financing health care services was then apportioned to the respective *obras sociales*. This measure had the effect of making the system of resource collection and allocation more transparent, clearly establishing the number of beneficiaries, and facilitating the control of evasion. In 1993, further advances were made on the reform policies in an attempt to solve two problems associated with the *obras sociales*. The first was related to the obligation imposed on workers to pay their health security contributions to the *obra social* associated with their particular trade union. In the view of the proponents of reform, this mechanism ensured a "captive" clientele incapable of raising the quantity and quality of services supplied or organising a more efficient administration of resources. It was believed that generating a certain degree of competition between the *obras sociales* might stimulate a greater degree of efficiency in their management and lead to the concentration of many small institutions into a few large ones capable of generating an adequate risk pool. In this way, it was hoped to reduce the great differences between institutions as to numbers of beneficiaries and availability of resources, which are frequently alleged to be the source of inequality in terms of benefits.

The second critical factor was the growing proportion of beneficiaries of *obras sociales* who were compelled to seek health care from the public subsystem. This phenomenon related to financial difficulties that compelled the *obras sociales* to resort to extra payments (co-payments) for additional service coverage. At the same time, professionals dissatisfied with low remuneration from the *obras sociales* began to charge their patients an additional fee at the time of service delivery. This extra fee was too much for some low-income beneficiaries, who were forced to resort to the free public services. Surveys of several general public hospitals revealed that 30–50% of their patients actually had insurance, even though the hospitals recovered only a negligible fraction of their costs from insurers. Of *obras sociales* members who were hospitalized in 1994, 5% reported that they relied on public health services, frequently without cost recovery. The adoption of new mechanisms that would allow hospitals and health centres to receive payment for their services has by and large been accepted, as it is believed that this will help alleviate their deficits and increase their cash flows.

Proposal backed by the World Bank

The Programmemea de Apoyo a la Reforma del Sistema de *Obras sociales* (PARSOS, programmeme in support of reform of the *Obras sociales* system), is backed by the World Bank and does not differ in concept from the strategy adopted by the government. Rather, it seeks to promote certain mechanisms. These have been listed in a recent publication by the Ministerio de Trabajo y Seguridad Social de la Nación (MTSS, ministry of labour and social security) as follows:

- introduce competition into the financial market, avoid risk selection;
- reassign resources from the Fondo Solidario de Redistribución (FSR, solidarity redistribution fund) strictly on the basis of income collected and risks per beneficiary;
- develop an effective regulatory framework;
- develop insurance institutions that are competitive,

transparent, and accountable, to protect consumers' rights; and

— provide financial and technical assistance to the *obras sociales* and the Programmemea de Atención Médica Integral (PAMI, comprehensive health care programmeme)http://archive.idrc.ca/books/focus/923/s2c02.htm - _ftn2, to enable them to increase their efficiency, balance their accounts, and comply with new norms and regulations.

The project also contemplates the preparation of lists of *obras sociales* beneficiaries, based on information that can be obtained from the Dirección General Impositiva (DGI, general administration of taxes). The specific purpose of this is to determine the number and risk factors of beneficiaries and their dependents. This information is essential for allocating subsidies, for maintaining transparency in contracts with health care managers, and for collecting fees for services supplied by public hospitals. A proposal was also put forward to define a Programmemea Médico Obligatorio (PMO, basic services package), able to guarantee minimum coverage within budgetary restrictions. The Fondo de Reconversión de *Obras sociales* (FROS, *Obras sociales* reconversion fund), was created to facilitate reform of the *obras sociales*' management. This would include helping them balance their budgets, restructure their debts, rationalize personnel, improve their managerial and information capability, and sell off idle assets. Participation in the programmeme is voluntary, but to date 73 *obras sociales* representing 5 million beneficiaries have joined the programmeme.

Counter-Proposal by the Confederación General Del Trabajo

This proposal aims to rationalize the *obras sociales*

under the autonomous coordination of the Confederación General del Trabajo (CGT, general labour confederation), while retaining the existing institutional structure and without generating competition between institutions or giving in to World Bank directives. The first point of the proposal deals with the definition of a Programmemea Médico Obligatorio (PMO, basic services package), along the lines that were later adopted by Decree 492. Once the PMO is defined, the Administración Nacional del Seguro de Salud (ANSSAL, national health insurance administration) will subsidize organisations unable to finance its application because of lack of resources. Should an *obra social* be unable to comply with the PMO due to misappropriation of funds, excessive management costs, inefficiency, noncompliance with quality standards, service irregularity, or any other cause detrimental to its function, ANSSAL has the power to merge it with another *obra social*. The Fondo Solidario de Redistribución (FSR, solidarity redistribution fund), would not only compensate organisations receiving insufficient resources, but would also aid in such processes as staff restructuring, negotiating with suppliers, upgrading equipment and facilities, and canceling current liabilities through loans. An important difference between the CGT project and the PARSOS project supported by the World Bank concerns distribution of subsidies by the FSR. In the CGT's proposal, the subsidy bears no relation to individual contributions by entitled beneficiaries, but is related instead to the average income per beneficiary of the *obra social*.

Implementation: Dispositions Regarding Social Security Institutions and Their Relations with Service Suppliers

The succession of government dispositions intended to give the reform a legislative framework illustrates to some degree the political conflict we have touched upon. Efforts to deregulate the *obras sociales* came one after the other without really being put into effect, the result of clashes that go beyond the bounds of the health sector. The following paragraphs contain a synthesis of the health reform legislation that has been approved.

Decree 9/93 (7 January 1993)

Decree 9 of 1993 sets out the guidelines for reform. It establishes, within certain limits, freedom of choice for affiliates to *obras sociales*. Named beneficiaries are entitled to choose between the system's component institutions and to change their affiliation once a year. The decree also establishes that the Ministerio de Salud y Acción Social de la Nación (MSAS, ministry of health and social action) will determine which basic services each *obra social* must deliver, and that the Administración Nacional del Seguro de Salud (ANSSAL, national health insurance administration), will cover the difference between contributions received and the actual cost of the services delivered.

The decree also undertakes to reform relations between *obras sociales* and providers of services through the following dispositions:

- The *obras sociales* are given freedom to contract with providers of services, without restriction as to scheduled fees, thus introducing price competition between health care suppliers.
- The *obras sociales* are forbidden to contract with institutions responsible for issuing professional licenses or limiting the right of their members to contract directly. This disposition excludes from the market those agents that have traditionally controlled the offer under oligopolistic conditions, that is, the professional associations.

— Contracts signed between *obras sociales* and providers shall contain criteria for categorizing and accrediting such providers, with the purpose of optimizing quality in health care.

— The *obras sociales* shall pay public hospitals for the services provided to their beneficiaries. This disposition is completed by Decree 578/93 regulating the *hospitales de autogestión* (self-managed hospitals). Self-managed hospitals are public hospitals that are empowered to manage their own resources independently of their respective jurisdictions (provincial or municipal) once they have complied with certain conditions stipulated in the decree. These hospitals will be discussed more fully in the section dealing with changes in the public sector.

Policies Reducing Employers' Contributions

The financial feasibility of the social security health system was threatened by the introduction of measures aimed at reducing the cost of labour by reducing employers' contributions to benefits. In March 1994, Decree 2.609 established that contributions for certain benefits could be reduced by different percentages, depending on geographical region. The effect on the funding of *obras sociales* was not uniform, revealing the incidence of other factors, particularly macro-level policies, on different sectors of economic activity. It should be noted that policies reducing employers' contributions underwent successive advances and setbacks in accordance with various levels of taxation and other variables at the macro level.

Decree 292/95 (14 August 1995)

Decree 292 has two objectives, to reduce excessive labour costs and assure the functioning of social security programmemes. This decree reinstated the reduction of contributions for those employers already benefiting under decree 722/25, and extended the privilege to all sectors of economic activity. In an attempt to make this reduction in labour costs compatible with basic health coverage for all, the decree guaranteed all *obras sociales* a minimum of US $30 (since 1991, 1 Argentine peso = US $1) per named beneficiary. Should an *obra social* collect less than this, the Fondo Solidario de Redistribución (FSR, solidarity redistribution fund), through the Administración Nacional del Seguro de Salud (ANSSAL, national health insurance administration), will grant a subsidy to make up the difference. For persons over 60 years old, the guaranteed amount per beneficiary is US $36. The resolution is important, not only because it guarantees minimum coverage and begins to recognize different risk levels, but also because it puts an end to the arbitrary distribution of subsidies on the part of the ANSSAL, a distribution that was historically motivated by political considerations.

Decree 492/95 (22 September 1995)

Decree 492/95 was motivated by pressure from trade unions opposed to the reduction of employers' contributions. Its main objective is to define a package of services that each *obra social* must guarantee its beneficiaries, and to ensure that each *obra social* has sufficient funding to provide such services. The resolution calls for the Ministerio de Salud y Acción Social de la Nación (MSAS, ministry of health and social action) and the Confederación General del Trabajo (CGT, general labour confederation) to designate a commission to be entrusted with establishing the package of services and setting the rules for its application. Also, the Decree raises the minimum guaranteed contribution to US $40 per beneficiary. Once the package has been approved, an *obra social* that finds itself unable to finance it has 60 days in which to propose a merger with one or more other organisations. Otherwise, the Administración Nacional del Seguro de Salud (ANSSAL, national health insurance administration) has the power to order a compulsory merger.

Unification of Jurisdictions — Superintendencia de Seguros de Salud

In December 1996, Decree 1615 took steps to rationalize policies. Its dispositions established the merger of different organisations having jurisdiction over the social security system, and created a new decentralized organisation, the Superintendencia de Seguros de Salud (SSS, superintendence of health insurance), dependent on the Ministerio de Salud y Acción Social de la Nación (MSAS, ministry of health and social action). The new state agency was administratively, economically, and financially autonomous, and was to be in charge of supervising, monitoring, and controlling agents' integration with the national health insurance system. Specific provisions make the SSS responsible for verifying compliance with the basic health services package; the Programmemea Nacional de Garantía de Calidad (national quality guarantee programmeme); the norms concerning self-managed hospitals; and the right of workers to chose their own *obra social*.

Reform of the Public Subsystem: Decentralisation of the Hospital System— Transfer of hospitals

Since the mid-1950s, several policies have gone part way toward transferring public health services from the national jurisdiction to the provinces. These transfers of health institutions were based on fiscal criteria, and did not go hand in hand with any mechanism for financial compensation, or any impetus toward improving service quality. Beginning in the 1990s, new decentralisation policies were set in motion, resulting in the transfer of 20 hospitals and some specialized institutions and social programmemes to the provincial level. Once again, the guiding motive was financial. With few exceptions, the decentralisation process from the national to the provincial level was not completed by transfers from the latter to the municipalities. In several cases, however, the provincial systems themselves developed a high degree of centralisation, although the outcomes varied by province due to different conditions. The nation has created hospitals endowed from their origin with a legislative structure that permits their decentralisation to the microeconomic unit (hospital) level. These are highly complex hospitals possessing, for example, the power to formulate budgets and set salaries, similarto the self-managed hospitals created and regulated under Decree 578/93.

Decree 578/93 (1 April 1993)

This decree created a national register of self-managed hospitals (Registro Nacional de Hospitales de Autogestión) and made it compulsory for *obras sociales*, mutual aid societies, and prepaid insurance schemes to pay for services received by their beneficiaries from public health facilities. To be eligible for incorporation into this system, hospitals were required to fulfill the following conditions:

- comply with all basic requirements established under the national quality programmeme, and be authorized and categorized by a competent authority;
- receive funding from the applicable jurisdiction on the basis of production, efficiency, and type of population served; and
- supplement their incomes with fees-for-services from persons able to pay, and with funds from contracts signed with private health-insurance companies, mutual aid societies, and *obras sociales*.

Extra-budgetary revenues thus received are to be

administered directly by the self-governing hospital. The hospitals were also authorized to use resources originating from the sale of services to create a structure of incentives based on recognition of productivity and staff efficiency, with a view to improving their administration. The future introduction of mechanisms for subsidizing demand was suggested, paving the way for the creation of public health insurance. Experience acquired to date has been limited to a few institutions, and the outcome has not been uniform. In some cases, the enrolment of patients with coverage has excluded or limited the access of poor people to the system; in other cases, that risk has been explicitly removed through administrative mechanisms that effectively prevent discrimination. In any event, the additional resources obtained in this way are not great when considered as a percentage of the total budgets of these institutions.

Throughout the 1990s, three phenomena concerning the decentralisation of the hospital system occurred simultaneously:

— The last of the national public hospitals was transferred to the provinces, achieving a decentralisation that was merely administrative in its aims.

— The provincial health systems were reconfigured, with some centralisation at the provincial level, but generally favouring decentralisation toward the municipalities, thus giving rise to a heterogeneous set of provincial situations.

— A certain degree of microeconomic decentralisation to the hospital level occurred in the form of the self-managed hospitals.

Evaluation: Effectiveness of Reform — The Underlying Political Conflict

It must be admitted that the effect of these measures on the existing system was small. One of the cornerstones of reform, deregulation of affiliation to the *obras sociales*, was blocked by firm opposition from the Confederación General del Trabajo (CGT, general labour confederation) Trade-union leaders defended maintenance of the status quo, chiefly because the financial resources of the *obras sociales* were an important source of economic and political power for them. Moreover, they had reason to believe that the labour movement may lose control of the system or be reduced to managing the portion with access to the fewest resources. Once freedom of choice between *obras sociales* came into effect, the door would be opened for competition with private insurance associations. It was feared that the latter would be able to attract affiliation from the higher-income stratum of the unionized population. The fact that reform decrees are issued at intervals of 2 years or so is linked with cycles of improvement and deterioration in the relations between the government and labour leaders. In more than a few instances, the existing system of *obras sociales* was allowed to continue in exchange for approval of other measures that the government deemed more important to the reform programmeme. On the other hand, the other pillar of reform — liberalisation of contractual measures affecting supply and demand of services — has had a significant impact on the greater part of the country. One has to ask, however, whether this is a consequence of reform measures or a movement initiated by entrepreneurs who have better opportunities elsewhere in view of financial crisis in social security. This point will be developed in the next section. Thus, a paradoxical situation has arisen whereby deregulation favours the competitiveness of the supplier as a result of fragmented demand, in the form of the survival of a number *obras sociales* controlling different levels of resources.

In 1995, several events affected the decision to push ahead with deregulation of the *obras sociales*, and revived the conflict with the CGT. The first of these was the Mexican crisis in December 1994, whose repercussions caused an upheaval in the Argentine financial system that lasted several months and prompted a new vote of confidence in the Convertibility Programmeme. A second event was the beginning of a recessionary phase in the economic cycle that highlighted the difficulty of controlling public spending and awakened well-grounded fears of a fiscal imbalance capable of threatening the monetary stability achieved earlier. Economic leaders stressed the need to deepen state reform and, to this end, to resolve outstanding questions concerning relations between the national and provincial governments, and between the state and the trade unions. As a step forward in the matter, negotiations were held with the World Bank spurred on by the need to achieve efficiency in the administration of expenditures. In the second half of 1996, talks between the government and union leaders deteriorated as a result of the Executive's decision to urge parliamentary sanction of the Leyes de Flexibilización Laboral, (labour flexibility laws). The CGT found all means of dialogue with the government blocked, and two general strikes were launched. The strikes received considerable public support given the government's loss of popularity due to its inability to reactivate the economy, to reverse staggering unemployment figures, to curb public spending or to control numerous cases of corruption and waste. The government continued its drive to make labour relations more flexible and at the same time set deadlines for the deregulation of the *obras sociales*. Since January 1,1997, beneficiaries have been able to choose their *obra social*.

Social Bases of the Conflict — New and Old Actors in the Health Sector

Contemporary analyses of health reform emphasize the study of national cases, using conceptual and methodological schemes for comparative analysis. Also, the perspective frequently shifts from a consideration of the state's form and functions to a preoccupation with relationships between state and society viewed as social constructions, that is, the result of historical processes. Attempts to explain the peculiarities exhibited by reform policies in each context thus focus on the political and institutional forms that represent interests and construct political consensus. In this way, the processes of policy formulation and application cease to be considered the result of rationalizing instances, but rather the result of dynamic processes between actors. These dynamic processes explain the formulation and reformulation of power relationships peculiar to the health sector and stemming from the agreements, alliances, clashes, and confrontations between its chief actors and, in particular, from the identities they build around the cohesion and legitimisation of the interests that they represent. Actors can be defined as:

> those individuals or groups occupying a strategic position in the decision-making system, and who are responsible, in the policy-forming process, for the functions of articulation of the cognitive field and the power field. In their role as mediators, it is they who define the issues of debate and the intellectual framework in which negotiations, alliances and conflicts sustaining decision-making take place." (Pierre Muller, taken from Merhy 1992, p. 46)

In the Argentine health services sector, the politically relevant actors have been, until very recently, large associations representing particular interests: the labour organisations, and the two large federations representing individual professionals and private hospitals, respectively.

To understand the changes in process, one must remember that competition between the political parties and these associations has been a relevant feature in Argentine politics since the 1940s. However, the last decade has seen the gradual weakening of the system by which associations represent their interests before the state. This is particularly noticeable in the changes that have come about in the relationship between the suppliers and users of services. Political analysts associate the weakening of corporate power with economic deregulation policies and with the decision to allow the rules of the marketplace greater play in the field of productive activity (Sidicaro 1995). To understand the weakening of the corporations at a time of strong state influence on the economy, it must be borne in mind that policies aimed at opening up the economy have had different effects on different sectors, and this has precluded the possibility of each of the traditional corporations presenting a united front. This is not to say that power relationships have dissolved as a consequence of competition in the marketplace. Rather, economic interests will now be represented before the state through lobbying practices, which, once adapted to some of the traditional features of Argentine political culture, will find new ways to increase clients. This is another of the features characterizing the new system of alliances in the health sector. The process was evident in corporations representing private hospitals even before contracting freedom between financing agencies and suppliers of health services was established. Faced with the financial crisis in the *obras sociales*, the institutions best able to compete began to offer more favourable contract conditions — in terms of costs and financial risks — to the *obras sociales*, either singly or collectively, thus giving rise to the first providers' networks. The weakening of the Confederación General del Trabajo (CGT, general labour confederation), manifested itself differently, though it surely had the same origin. The leadership of the trade unions was affected in the 1990s by three interrelated processes:

— structural transformations that modified the composition of the labour force and increased the heterogeneity of wages and employment;
— changes in the political culture of negotiating work conditions that have resulted in a general drive toward collective agreements by company as opposed to labour specialty, which was the foundation of much of the trade unions' power; and
— antagonisms that have arisen between labour leaders adopting divergent positions with regard to the liberalisation policies pushed by a government that purports to share their Peronist ideals but has relinquished, one by one, the traditional banners of the movement.

In this context, the relationship between the government and the trade unions is being continually redefined. Control of the *obras sociales* is frequently used as a bargaining chip in the face of other issues that are perceived as more pressing to — or less reconcilable with — the reform process being carried out by the Ministerio de Economía de la Nación (ministry of the economy). In this way, the structural features that would redefine the relationship are continually subject to changes based on matters of the moment. Another weighty factor at the political level is the power struggle for the presidential succession in 1999, and the apparent intention of the candidate most likely to win to reinstate the traditional alliances of the Peronist movement, with Menem's support. Thus, under Menemism, the labour movement has fragmented, giving rise to two groups opposed to the CGT: the Movimiento de los Trabajadores Argentinos (Argentine workers movement) and the Congreso de los Trabajadores

Argentinos (Argentine workers' congress). However, some components of the labour movement, those closest to the government's liberal tendencies, have radically transformed their organisations into what has been called sindicalismo de negocios or business unionism. Changes in the union movement go beyond the weakening the negotiating capability of the CGT, however. The labour leaders best able to profit from the privatisation of public enterprises or the deregulation of services production have begun to incorporate entrepreneurial functions into their traditional activities The following are examples of positioning by trade unions in the face of changes affecting their place in the scheme of things: management of *Programmemeas de Propiedad Participada*, shared ownership programmemes, in privatized public enterprises; organisation of micro-enterprises for petroleum prospecting and electric power generation; and participation in companies that administer retirement funds or health care management organisations. The CGT's opposition to the deregulation of the *obras sociales* did not therefore come about in a context of institutional paralysis. Despite confrontation with the government at the political level, a large number of them have begun to develop a new managerial capability with a view to adapting to the new scenario. At present, their strategies are aimed in three main directions.

1. An important group of *obras sociales* — 73 institutions representing about 5 million beneficiaries — have opted for the advantages offered by the *Programmemea de Reconversión del Sector Salud* (health sector reform programmeme), financed by the World Bank.
2. A second group — made up of smaller entities unable to form an adequate risk pool individually — have begun merging or forming federations. In the first

case, that of a merger, the result is a new *obra social*. In the second case, a federation, the entities retain their legal individuality but pool the collection and administration of their financial resources.

3. Lastly, some *obras sociales*, individually or in groups of three or more, are associating with local or foreign companies to form a new association, under the legal form of a stock company or something similar, to act as health care management agencies for all their beneficiaries, and to provide an alternative in a deregulated situation.

To further complicate the situation, since 1994 of multinational capital of varied origin to the health services system. Companies such as Amil, the Excel Group, The Principal, Provida, Swiss Medical Group and others have acquired local health service institutions or have formed joint ventures for the future management of such institutions. They have also entered the field of private insurance, or have acted as consulting agencies dedicated to improving the management of financing institutions, individual providers, or providers' networks. Another field that they have entered is health services administration, by associating with or absorbing existing institutions, or by creating new ones. The crisis that affected all levels of society throughout the 1980s, culminating in the hyperinflation of 1989, signaled the depletion of some of the country's fundamental institutions. Recovery in the 1990s came about partly as a result of rethinking the logic governing them. At the economic level, this was reflected in the results of the policies for liberalizing the economy and, in particular, one of the most effective instruments of these policies, the Convertibility Plan. At the political level this led to state reform, which has not yet been completed.

The health services system could not remain untouched by the financial crisis and the transformations that followed. In the public sector, the reduction of fiscal spending aggravated long-standing conditions of decay and decadence. These public services, intended for the poor population, found their clientele increased by contingents of "new poor": members of the lower and middle classes suffering the consequences of unemployment, informal labour, self-employment, and precarious labour relations. The *obras sociales* were affected by the same processes, through a decrease in the population covered and an attendant reduction of contributions; evasion on the part of contributors; and increased disagreement within the system as to the distribution of funds. To these factors originating outside the health sector, must be added others equally or more important. They relate to longstanding deficiencies or distortions in the health services organisation, including: extreme fragmentation and heterogeneity in the *obras sociales*; the reluctance of the state organisations concerned to put them in order; an overloading of public services due to the demands of those with insufficient coverage; the predominance of the private sector in the supply of services; the existence of methods of payment that encouraged oversupply and overcharging; and the expansion of installed capacity and a supply of technology that exceeded the ability to pay. All of these were manifestations of the exhaustion of the organisational mode prevalent up to that time.

The state's response was expressed both in terms of freedom to sign contracts and deregulation in the area of social security, and in terms of localisation and decentralisation — at institutional and territorial levels — in the policies applied to the public sector. Contracting freedom between financing organisations and providers of health services was quickly adopted by the private sector in response to an oversupply of services. The corporations traditionally predominant in this sector quickly lost the oligopoly that they had enjoyed through control of contracts with the *obras sociales*. New forms of intermediaries such as service management agencies, transient company mergers, and suppliers' networks undertook the management of risk contracts incorporating per-capita methods of payment. New forms of services supply were incorporated and cost-containment strategies that placed family physicians or general practitioners in a "gatekeeper" role, were tried out. Financing possibilities were enlarged through the expansion of private insurance organisations. On the demand side, reform encountered obstacles that were harder to surmount because they were rooted in conditions outside the health sector, mainly the confrontational relationship between the state and the trade unions that had existed since the beginning of the 1950s. Interest on the part of reformers — part of the government and the World Bank — centered on eliminating the "captive population" of the *obras sociales* by allowing union members freedom of choice between institutions administering social security contributions. In this way, it was hoped to stimulate competition, to generate incentives to reduce administration costs, and to offer better quality health care. The refusal of the Confederación General del Trabajo (CGT, general labour confederation), which uses the *obras sociales* as a bargaining chip with the government whenever discussions arise concerning production policies, employment policies, or the survival of leaders' privileges, has blocked the application of the reform decrees during the last 3 years.

The process has been more complex within the associations of suppliers, because these are not groupings of business organisations, but groupings of institutions having mixed political and trade-union bases. Their adaptation to the new contracting conditions has been accomplished by means of different strategies, such as the formation of private insurance companies, the purchase of private hospitals, the installation of ambulatory diagnostic and surgical centres, and the introduction of the associations into existing supplier networks. In this way, they have attempted to assure their members a place in the supply of services.

Private hospitals, *obras sociales*' hospitals, and to a lesser degree, independent professionals continue to hold a predominant place in the structure of the health services system, particularly in matters relating to the regulation of supply conditions; the incorporation of technology; changes in the way services are organised, and in the control of supply conditions. Now, however, the regulation of supply conditions is no longer accomplished through a centralized entity guaranteeing equal access to demand by all members of the corporation, but rather through the dynamic interplay of business competition in quest of contracts with the *obras sociales*.

Bibliography

Bates DW, Spell N, Cullen DJ, Burdick E, Laird N, Petersen LA, et al. The costs of adverse drug events in hospitalized patients. Adverse Drug Events Prevention Study Group. *JAMA* 1997; 277:307-311.

Bowman L, Carlstedt BC, Black CD. Incidence of adverse drug reactions in adult medical inpatients. *Can J Hosp Pharm* 1994; 47:209-216.

Bradshaw KE, Gardner RM, Pryor TA. Development of a computerized laboratory alerting system. *Comput Biomed Res* 1989; 22:575-587.

Classen DC, Pestotnik SL, Evans RS, Lloyd JF, Burke JP. Adverse drug events in hospitalized patients. Excess length of stay, extra costs, and attributable mortality. *JAMA* 1997; 277:301-306.

Cullen DJ, Bates DW, Small SD, Cooper JB, Nemeskal AR, Leape LL. The incident reporting system does not detect adverse drug events: a problem for quality improvement. *Jt Comm J Qual Improv* 1995; 21:541-548.

Cullen DJ, Sweitzer BJ, Bates DW, Burdick E, Edmondson A, Leape LL. Preventable adverse drug events in hospitalized patients: a comparative study of intensive care and general care units. *Crit Care Med* 1997; 25:1289-1297.

Hutchinson TA, Flegel KM, Kramer MS, Leduc DG, Kong HH. Frequency, severity and risk factors for adverse drug reactions in adult out-patients: a prospective study. *J Chronic Dis* 1986; 39:533-542.

Johnson JA, Bootman JL. Drug-related morbidity and mortality. A cost-of-illness model. *Arch Intern Med* 1995; 155:1949-1956.

Kellaway GS, McCrae E. Intensive monitoring for adverse drug effects in patients discharged from acute medical wards. *N Z Med J* 1973; 78:525-528.

Kuperman GJ, Teich JM, Tanasijevic MJ, Ma'Luf N, Rittenberg E, Jha A, et al. Improving response to critical laboratory results with automation: results of a randomized controlled trial.

McDonald CJ. Use of a computer to detect and respond to clinical events: its effect on clinician behavior. *Ann Intern Med* 1976; 84:162-167.

Raschke RA, Gollihare B, Wunderlich TA, Guidry JR, Leibowitz AI, Peirce JC, et al.

Index